FAILUI

MW01269129

"In the fall of 1988, I was a rookie in the MCPD Academy class. While out on a training run with my classmates, we were joined by this incredibly fit SWAT member (Jeff Nyce) who began to run next to us for encouragement. Throughout the remainder of my thirty-year career with MCPD, I never met an individual more consistent, determined, or focused on the quest for excellence than Jeff Nyce. As his commander in the Special Operations Division, I found it apparent that the fervor and love Sergeant Jeff Nyce's officers had for him was never demanded but earned through unwavering leadership in his character, conduct, and commitment. When the division was not responding to life safety missions within the field, Jeff was constantly asking the 'what if' questions internally to ensure we were prepared to face the next more complicated situation that none of us had ever met. Through his visionary leadership and team-first approach, we never failed. I am grateful that countless readers will now be able to share this gem of a man through a brief glimpse into his life. Even when Jeff was on death's doorstep fighting a terminal situation that would have devoured the average human being, he not only defied logic but continued to inspire the rest of us through his grit and upbeat resolve while still focused on others. Upon reading this book, you will truly know what it means to live a committed life."

Chief of Police Darryl McSwain

The Maryland-National Capital Park Police

Montgomery County Division

Former Director, Special Operations Division

Montgomery County Department of Police, Maryland

"Jeff Nyce, while a great tactician and operator, is a true leader of men who was consistently committed to improving the effectiveness of his team and achieving the best outcomes during all operations no matter how simple or complex. In a unique way, Jeff always understood the superordinate goal of getting better and never celebrated the status quo. He understood the emerging challenges of events such as active-shooter and terrorist threats and had a unique focus on technology, training, and leadership. He is selfless, passionate, and committed, and he excelled in developing others, building trust, building alliances, and making certain he and his team were prepared for all foreseeable challenges, problems, and circumstances. He is one of the all-time best, not as much for what he accomplished but for how he touched and further developed our industry and the individuals and teams he interacted with throughout his career. This is a remarkable story and will serve as an inspiration to all who read his book."

Chief of Police Luther Reynolds
Charleston Police, South Carolina
Former Director, Special Operations Division
Montgomery County Department of Police, Maryland

FAILURE'S NOT AN OPTION

by

Jeff Nyce

With Richard Ziegfeld

Dedication

To my teammates on Montgomery County SWAT—brothers for life.

To my wife, Jayne, and my son, Lawrence.

Table of Contents

Table of Tables

Foreword: Brian Dillman

"Have to." "Will do." "All good." All are phrases I have heard my very dear friend and former counterpart say hundreds of times over the past twenty-two years. Although these may seem like simple phrases, they are the words that define the way in which Jeff Nyce tackles every aspect of his life. This book, titled *Failure's Not an Option,* illustrates Jeff Nyce's life mantra.

My friendship with Jeff began in 1997 when I was selected to be a member of the Montgomery County Police Department's SWAT Team. At that time, Jeff had already been a member of the team for thirteen years. Over the next twenty-two years, I would have the distinct pleasure and honor to be mentored by Jeff; supervise the Montgomery County SWAT Team together; become the closest of friends; become the godfather of his only child and son, Lawrence Todd; and witness his ongoing battle with cancer.

Jeff and I conducted several thousand tactical operations together. For Jeff, the mission always came first. He was meticulous in his training, preparation, planning, and execution of all aspects of the job. He put everything he had into everything he did. Even more impressive was the fact that Jeff always found the strengths of his teammates and mentored and encouraged them. He always knew what was at stake in every mission. He knew that to never fail, every member of the team had to be prepared and put in the best position to help the team win.

To illustrate Jeff's perspective on SWAT missions, he often used this analogy. The 2007 New England Patriots went 16-0 during the regular season but lost in the Super Bowl. To most, this was viewed as a very successful football season. They won far more games that season than any other NFL team, but they lost the biggest game of their season. Conversely, for a SWAT team, every operation is a Super Bowl. A loss is a catastrophic failure. A loss for a SWAT team means an innocent civilian or a fellow officer is injured or, worse, killed. A SWAT team may not lose. Failure's not an option. During Jeff's tenure on the team, we were undefeated. We never lost! This was in large part due to Jeff's "never quit, have to, mission first" mindset.

Up until 2012, I had primarily seen Jeff's mantra play out in his professional but not his personal life. This all changed in September of 2012, only one month after the passing of Jeff's mom, Sandy, from ovarian cancer, when he shared with me the fact that he had been diagnosed with multiple myeloma and cardiac amyloidosis.

I have now watched Jeff battle his cancer and amyloidosis for the past eight years. The same "have to, never quit, never fail, never give up" mindset has enabled Jeff to defy all medical odds. Jeff has made medical history and has amazed and mystified doctors across the globe.

Although Jeff may have surprised those in the medical profession who do not know him well, he has not surprised me. In 2015, Jeff suffered a stroke. I had recently read Laura Hillenbrand's book *Unbroken* about Louis Zamperini and took a copy of it to Jeff to read. I had inscribed this note in it before giving it to him: "Jeff, I thought it was only appropriate that I give a true warrior a book to read about another warrior. You are the strongest individual I have ever known both physically and mentally. This book reminds me of you. You are my real-life Louie. This stroke is nothing more than another one of the many obstacles that have been put in your path that you have defeated. Keep your chin up, continue to fight and persevere like you always do. I love you, my brother. God bless, Brian."

Failure's Not an Option provides insight about the perspective of a modern-day warrior whose mindset has always conquered any obstacle—without fail—because failure has never been an option for Jeff in either his professional or personal life.

Lieutenant Brian Dillman

Deputy Director of Special Operations Division

Montgomery County Department of Police, Maryland

Preface

When I was struck down at the height of my SWAT career with two life-threatening diseases and retired in 2014, I lost my sense of identity. SWAT was my passion, and I was at the top of my game when illnesses forced me into an unanticipated retirement. I suddenly found myself unable to work at any level. I attempted to work the first two years after retirement but could only manage four days a year. The effects of daily, long-term, heavy chemotherapy treatment; a stroke; and other medical complications had made the struggle to survive too great, so any employment was out of the question.

At a loss, I started to reflect on my career and the medical journey that followed. Soon, I was writing down my thoughts and experiences and focused primarily on the facts. I documented these events when I felt up to it, though it was unpredictable how I would feel on any given day. This circumstance made progress slow and erratic, but it afforded me great flexibility because I was not bound to a schedule that a traditional job requires.

Three years later, after I had accumulated a lengthy "memoir," I met Richard Ziegfeld, who had a background in editing and writing. We had some discussions and jointly decided to work on publishing the memoir. During this phase, we focused on three aspects of the memoir:

1. We expanded the scope to include many more incidents.

2. I reached out to teammates, family, and medical professionals who enriched the stories with new detail and insights.

3. Through dialogue with Richard, I moved from focusing mostly on facts to add introspective insights and feelings.

This new focus on writing has helped me recover my sense of identity and gain a renewed sense of purpose. I have always been a goal-driven individual. This project provided me with a new goal: to publish a memoir that I hope others will find both intriguing and inspirational.

Table of Acronyms

Acronym	Definition
AL	Amyloid Light-Chain
ALP	Alkaline Phosphatase
ALT	Alanine Aminotransferase Test
APC	Armored Personnel Carriers
AR	Armalite Rifle
AST	Aspartate Aminotransferase
ATF	Bureau of Alcohol, Tobacco, Firearms, and Explosives
CRNP	Certified Registered Nurse Practitioner
DHS	Department of Homeland Security
DMSO	Dimethyl Sulfoxide
DSWAT	Decentralized Special Weapons and Tactics
ECM	Electronic Counter Measures
ERT	Emergency Response Team
FAA	Federal Aviation Administration
HEPA	High-Efficiency Particulate Air
HRT	Hostage Rescue Team
IAT	Immediate Action Team
ICE	Immigration and Customs Enforcement
ICU	Intensive Care Unit
IED	Improvised Explosive Device

Acronym	Definition
IID	Improvised Incendiary Device
IRA	Irish Republican Army
JOC	Joint Operations Center
MCPD	Montgomery County Police Department
MRI	Magnetic Resonance Image
MSP	Maryland State Police
NCR	National Capital Region
NHLBI	National Heart, Lung, and Blood Institute
NIH	National Institutes of Health
OEE	Office of Export Enforcement
PBIED	Person-Borne Improvised Explosive Device
PCAT	Police Community Action Team
PCP	Phencyclidine
PO3	Police Officer 3
PT	Physical Training
REPR	Rapid Engagement Precision Rifles
RSP	Render Safe Procedures
SOD	Special Operations Division
SRT	Special Response Team
SWAT	Special Weapons and Tactics
UMMC	University of Maryland Medical Center
V&I	Vice and Intelligence

Introduction

In the thirty years I spent in Special Weapons and Tactics (SWAT), I participated in some of the most highly publicized events in law enforcement history, which generated national and even international attention, including the takedown of the DC snipers. I was also involved in a hostage rescue incident by a lone-wolf domestic terrorist who the FBI determined was "the first suicide bomber with hostages in the United States" at the Discovery Headquarters Building in Silver Spring, Maryland, and the capture of a violent group of serial bank robbers featured on John Walsh's *America's Most Wanted*. These events and the 4,500 raids and barricades I participated in over my career helped to prepare me for the life-threatening medical incidents that transpired beginning in 2010 and continue to today.

At the height of my career as a SWAT commander, I was struck down by two diseases that at the time were deemed terminal with no available cure: multiple myeloma cancer and cardiac amyloidosis. Doctors told me I had less than two years to live—at best. I prepared for what would be the greatest fight of my life. A career in SWAT had trained me for this fight, with its quarterly fitness tests, numerous high-risk operations, and the mindset to persist against seemingly insurmountable odds.

I overcame many obstacles, including "coding" in 2013 during a stem-cell transplant that required chest compressions and saline to bring me back to life and then a stroke precipitated in 2015 by the chemotherapy I was undergoing to forestall the myeloma and amyloidosis.

I applied the same expectations that I had of the SWAT Team to myself, always telling the team, "Never complain, never quit, and the mission comes first. Failure's not an option as it relates to the mission." My mission is simple: survive.

Eight years have passed since my initial diagnosis, and I am still alive and in remission, and by all medical accounts, I have defied the odds.

This memoir consists of three elements: high-profile SWAT operations; my medical journey; and lessons on fitness, diet, and drug routines that have helped me manage these medical obstacles and improve my quality of life.

My hope is that by sharing these incidents in SWAT and the medical odyssey that followed, I can help others manage their illnesses, improve their quality of life, and enjoy (directly or vicariously) the high-speed SWAT experiences and the medical risks that my medical team took for me.

Jeff Nyce
Montgomery County, Md.
January 2020

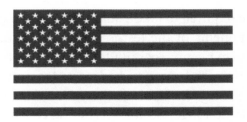

1. DC Snipers

"We started as a team and finished as a team"

I woke up in the morning feeling very fatigued. My body ached, in particular my bones, muscles, and joints in the back, trapezius, and shoulders. I was also experiencing shortness of breath with any type of physical exertion. I had been experiencing these symptoms for about a year, and they had progressively gotten worse. For the last several months, I had strategically placed half a dozen ice packs on those parts of the body that hurt the most as I went to sleep at night. The ice packs were now scattered across the bed.

My future wife, Jayne, knew of my ailments and asked, "Honestly, how do you feel?" I said, "Honestly, I feel like I'm dying." Two years later, I would find out this perception was true.

I had attributed my ailments to my career. I was the SWAT commander for the Montgomery County Police Department (MCPD) in Maryland. The job was physically demanding, and we worked around the clock, averaging 200 raids/barricades a year. I often averaged three to four hours of sleep a night, which made me assume this was why I was so fatigued. I was fifty-three years old and recognized that my body didn't recover as quickly. Years of weight training, running, and wearing heavy body armor had taken a toll.

The shortness of breath greatly concerned me because I had always been a decent runner. Every three months as a member of the SWAT Team, officers are required to take a quarterly physical training (PT) test. One of the components of the test is a three-mile run that we had to complete in less than twenty-six minutes. At age fifty-two, I was running it in 20:30. Then over the last year, I had started to notice a huge increase in my times, and my legs felt like lead every time I ran. It was clear that in the future I would no longer be able to run the course in under twenty-six minutes, which meant I would no longer qualify for the SWAT Team.

SWAT was my passion. I had been a police officer for thirty-one years, with twenty-eight years in SWAT. The men on the team were my best friends, all highly motivated, skilled, athletic, smart, and driven. They are all men of honor and valor and have the utmost integrity. Being around such people elevated my own game, and each officer helped me become a better person.

These ailments prompted me to reflect on my career in SWAT. I had done thousands of raids and barricades, but one particular operation stood out above the others. In October of 2002, Lee Boyd Malvo and John Allen Muhammad terrorized the Washington metropolitan area, shooting thirteen people over a three-week period in the DC area. The search for the "snipers" became one of the largest manhunts in law enforcement history.

October 3, 2002, was the day that kicked off activity in Montgomery County, Maryland, which borders the northern side of the nation's capital. It occupies 500-plus square miles and has a population of one million. At 7:41 a.m., James Sonny Buchanan (age thirty-nine) was shot and killed while mowing the grass near the Colonial Dodge car dealership in a busy area of Rockville, Maryland. This shooting made it personal for every MCPD officer because the victim was the son of one of our retired officers.

A short time later in Montgomery County, Premakuar Walekar (fifty-four), a cab driver, was shot and killed at 8:12 a.m. while pumping gas at a Mobil service station in Aspen Hill, Maryland. The tragic shooting of Walekar made things more complicated for the police. At the time of his shooting, a funeral procession was en route to the Gate of Heaven Cemetery in Aspen Hill to bury Montgomery County Police Officer William Faust, who had died several days before of a heart attack. The shooting of Walekar took place only 400 yards from the cemetery. Officer Faust was a thirty-year veteran with many law enforcement ties throughout the region. He had been a motor officer most of his life (traffic specialist) and had assisted me in accident reconstruction early in my career as a rookie patrol officer. In attendance were hundreds of police officers from multiple jurisdictions as well as family and friends.

Although we knew of no link between the two shootings at this point, Commander of the 3rd District Station (and my former SWAT sergeant) Drew Tracy thought it would be prudent to protect the site. MCPD SWAT set up sniper positions around the cemetery, and numerous patrol officers deployed along the route in defensive positions. In addition, Tracy reached out to our neighboring jurisdiction, Prince George's County, for air support. Prince George's County has helicopters, so its officials provided a helicopter to escort and watch over the funeral motorcade as it made its way to the cemetery without incident. It was a hurried and uncomfortable burial because everyone present was aware of the recent shootings.

When the motorcade was making its way to the cemetery at 8:37 a.m., Sara Ramos (thirty-four) was shot and killed while sitting on a bench in front of a post office at the Leisure World Shopping Center just three miles north of the last shooting. Witnesses reported seeing a white box truck leaving the scene at a high rate of speed, and it was thought that the sound of shots had come from the proximity of the white box truck. This was the first vehicle lookout the police had in reference to the shootings. Those SWAT officers who were not assigned to the cemetery detail formed two-man teams and stopped every white box truck we saw.

Not long after that, at 9:58 a.m. in Kensington, Maryland, six miles from the last shooting, Lori Ann Lewis-Rivera (twenty-five) was shot and killed at a Shell gas station while she was vacuuming her van. Her two-year-old daughter was in the vehicle.

This alarming series of events involved four shootings in two hours.

All were one-shot, one-kill incidents, leading to speculation that we may be dealing with a sniper. All shootings occurred in busy, congested areas. I believed that whoever was doing these shootings wanted a fight, and I thought the bloodshed would continue that day until there was a shootout with the police. Then suddenly everything became very quiet. It was an eerie calm compared to the high-speed velocity experienced early on. SWAT continued to work into the evening, and then at 9:15 p.m., one-hundred feet inside the DC line from Montgomery County, Pascol Charlot (seventy-two) was shot and killed on the sidewalk. With the shooter still active, SWAT worked through the night and into the next day.

MCPD investigators soon determined that there had been two shootings that occurred the previous evening in our county that appeared to be related to the sniper phenomenon. At 5:00 p.m. the night before, a shot was fired through a plate-glass window at a Michaels arts and crafts store in Aspen Hill. A cashier reported feeling something hissing as the bullet passed. Fortunately, nobody was injured. The Michaels store was about 200 yards from the Gate of Heaven Cemetery, where Officer William Faust had been buried. Aspen Hill seemed to be a popular place for the shooter.

One hour later, at 6:04 p.m., James D. Martin (fifty-five) was shot and killed four miles away in the parking lot of the Shoppers Food Warehouse in the Glenmont Shopping Center. The shooter or shooters were brazen. One hundred yards across the street from where Martin was shot is the MCPD Fourth District Station, which had 150 officers assigned to it.

We sent two senior snipers to the scenes of all the shootings to gather intelligence and ascertain from where the shots were being fired. In particular, we wanted to determine if the shots were being taken from an elevated position. Upon completing the recon, the MCPD snipers concluded the shots were not being taken from an elevated position.

Early on, the Bureau of Alcohol, Tobacco, Firearms, and Explosives (ATF) began analyzing ballistic evidence. It soon determined that the shootings were related and that it was a .223-caliber firearm. The .223 caliber is most closely associated with the AR-15 (Armalite Rifle) that the military adopted and evolved into the M16 and various models thereafter. It is a high-velocity round with an effective range of 500 to 600 yards and is capable of penetrating some types of police body armor.

SWAT worked through the night and into the following day, when we expected it to start all over again. Everything was quiet. Instead, the snipers struck sixty miles south of our county in Fredericksburg, Virginia. Forty-three-year-old Caroline Seawell was shot in the lower back after shopping at a crafts store at a local mall. Fortunately, she survived the shooting.

The MCPD needed additional assets at all levels. Every day, hundreds of phone calls were received about suspicious persons, vehicles, and other data that required follow-up. Investigators were overwhelmed. The federal government brought in numerous resources (manpower and technology) at the investigative level: the FBI, ATF, U.S. Marshals Service, Secret Service, and others. They took over an entire commercial building next to the MCPD headquarters for their Joint Operations Center (JOC). They brought Rapid Start, a case information management system set up by the FBI to help keep track of the incredibly large volume of information. The feds brought much more in terms of technology and manpower to assist our investigators.

We also needed additional tactical assets. MCPD SWAT had a long-standing history with both the FBI Hostage Rescue Team (HRT) and the Maryland State Police (MSP) SWAT Team. On numerous occasions, our SWAT Team had been to FBI facilities in Quantico, Virginia. The FBI HRT provided us with training and use of its facilities. One of our former SWAT Team members was an FBI HRT leader. The MSP SWAT Team had always been there when we needed it. Both agencies provided us with additional tactical personnel. We were able to field two shifts of thirty, so that at any given moment we had thirty tactical officers on duty nearly twenty-four hours a day. A significant resource that the FBI and state teams provided was helicopters, assets we lacked. The FBI deployed sniper teams on its aircraft to provide overwatch and protection from above. The Montgomery County Sheriff's Department had a six-man Special Response Team (SRT) that supplemented us as well.

Initial discussion among the agencies focused on tactical command and control—that is, who would be in charge of a tactical incident with the agencies mixed and matched. We agreed that if a tactical incident occurred in Montgomery County, the MCPD SWAT Team would be the lead agency and that if a tactical incident occurred outside of Montgomery County, the FBI HRT would lead. The FBI federalized both MCPD and MSP SWAT Teams. This gave our SWAT Teams standard law enforcement powers outside our jurisdiction to include other states. If the FBI HRT wanted, it could bring SWAT officers from the MSP and MCPD to assist in tactical operations outside their normal jurisdictions.

The overall lead for the MCPD Task Force was Drew Tracy. When the shootings occurred, our agency was transitioning to a new radio system, which created some potential inter-agency communication problems. Commander Tracy came up with an idea that I first thought would be problematic but turned out to be brilliant. To overcome the radio issue, he wanted to mix and match the teams. He wanted one MCPD SWAT officer, one MSP SWAT officer, and one FBI HRT member in each vehicle. The concern I had was that as SWAT officers we all know tactics, but no two SWAT teams do things exactly the same way. Commander Tracy wanted all the SWAT officers in MCPD vehicles and MCPD SWAT officers driving. The concept was that all calls for service would come over the MCPD police radio, and the tactical officers from the three agencies would all hear the calls at the same time. Further, he wanted the MCPD officers driving because they knew the area best and could provide a quick, efficient response.

I was the MCPD SWAT Team leader on the night shift. In my unmarked Jeep Cherokee were First Sergeant Keith Runk (the MSP SWAT Team leader) and Chuck Pierce (the FBI HRT Team leader and supervisor). We were the command vehicle for the evening shift, and there were nine other three-man SWAT vehicles mixed and matched like ours, giving us thirty tactical operators. The first day we rode together, I recall telling Runk and Pierce that I believed we were going to be the ones that would get the snipers, meaning our agencies—FBI HRT, MSP SWAT, and MCPD SWAT. As fate would have it, all three of us would be on the Assault Team. My concerns about a mixed and matched team rapidly disappeared as we quickly jelled into one team, and our movements became second nature to one another, just as it would be with our own teammates.

We developed two types of proactive tactical responses to any sniper-related shooting incident: an in-county and an out-of-county response. If a shooting occurred in our county, the goal was to get one of our three-man SWAT vehicles on scene within two to three minutes. The on-scene SWAT unit would provide site security. We would create a concentric circle with a perimeter of three to five miles in all directions from the shooting site. All the traffic lights in Montgomery County operate on an automated system. Every traffic signal within the three- to five-mile radius would be put on flashing red. This would create a massive traffic jam and slow the egress of any suspects attempting to leave the crime scene. Plainclothes units would monitor the traffic at key points looking for any vehicle similar to one in a "lookout" or suspicious vehicles or persons.

Staged in proximity to the plainclothes units were our three-man SWAT vehicles. If we needed to stop and investigate a vehicle, SWAT would make the stop. At the same time, the FBI HRT helicopters would be overhead surveying the area and supporting the officers on the ground. Slowing the traffic gave police the ability to create choke points so that in some circumstances, we could stop, search, and investigate every vehicle.

If a shooting occurred outside of Montgomery County, every plainclothes and SWAT unit had a predetermined location to respond to. The idea was to monitor every point of entry into Montgomery County. Once again, officers would search for any similar vehicle wanted in a "lookout" or suspicious vehicles or persons entering the county. If we identified a vehicle of interest, a SWAT vehicle would make the stop with tactical support from HRT helicopters.

On any given day, dozens of phone calls would come into the Montgomery County 911 Emergency Center reporting suspicious persons, vehicles, or other information related to the snipers. In each instance, SWAT would investigate—e.g., clearing wood lines, searching buildings, and checking persons and vehicles. The team leaders would help coordinate the response of the three tactical agencies to these incidents.

The snipers invoked tremendous fear in the community everywhere. Gas stations had tarps draped at fuel pumps so that customers could not be seen as they pumped gas. Citizens could be seen running and zigzagging through the parking lot as they went to the grocery store. At the SWAT level, we were not sure if this was domestic terrorism or foreign terrorism related to Al- Qaeda because it was only one year after 9/11. Investigators followed up on all leads on both fronts.

Of great concern was the safety of schools. Early on, command made a decision to put MCPD officers at every school as they opened and closed. Principals cancelled all outdoor and after-school activities. Each day, as schools opened and closed, helicopters from the MSP and FBI hovered—low and loud—to give a strong presence.

Our neighboring jurisdiction, Prince George's County, had not experienced the early onslaught that we had: no shootings to date and so no upgraded police presence at its schools.

On October 7, at Benjamin Tasker Middle School in Bowie, Maryland, thirteen-year-old Iran Brown's aunt, Tanya Brown, was dropping him off at school. Iran was shot shortly after he exited the vehicle, and he fell to the ground. Tanya heard a shot and a scream and saw him lying on the ground. She backed the car up and could see blood on his shirt. Iran stood up and said he had been shot and climbed into the car. Brown immediately called 911 on her cell phone and drove to the Bowie Health Center, an emergency clinic. Her quick, decisive actions saved his life.

We were told after the suspects were in custody that this was supposed to be a mass shooting of kids. A school bus had pulled up in front of the school, preparing to unload students. An empty bus then pulled in front of the loaded bus, blocking the snipers' view and preventing what could have been a much greater tragedy. Poor Iran Brown simply happened to be a target of opportunity.

Shootings continued in Virginia. On October 9 at 8:10 p.m., Dean Harold Myers (fifty-three) was shot in the head and killed at the

Battlefield Sunoco in Manassas. Two days later at 9:28 a.m., Kenneth Bridges (also fifty-three) was shot and killed at the 4-Mile Fork Exxon in Spotsylvania County. Then on October 14 at 9:15 p.m. in Fairfax County, FBI analyst Linda Franklin (forty-seven) was shot in the head and killed in a Home Depot parking lot. She died in her husband's arms.

At the Franklin shooting, witnesses reported seeing a white van near where the sound of shots came from. The "lookout vehicle" for police went from a white box truck to a white van. A check through the Motor Vehicle Administration showed that there were more than 10,000 white vans registered in the DC region. We stopped hundreds of white vans in Montgomery County. For every vehicle we stopped, we used a tactic termed "position and call." From a position of cover from our own vehicle, we would call the occupants back to our location. From there we would pat them down for weapons. One officer would remain with the subjects, who would be seated on the curb while the other two officers went up and "cleared" the vehicle.

We did this hundreds of times with no complaints from the public because people understood the magnitude of the situation. Early on, it became apparent that law enforcement was stopping some of the same white vans over and over. To alleviate this problem, we placed small identifiable stickers on the rear tags of those white vans that law enforcement had already stopped.

On October 19 at 8:00 p.m., Jeffrey Hopper (thirty-seven) was shot in the abdomen in Ashland, Virginia. His wife saved his life by applying pressure to the wound until fire and rescue arrived.

Conrad Johnson (thirty-five), a bus driver for Montgomery County's Ride On transit system, was shot at 5:56 a.m. on October 22 while parked just off Connecticut Avenue in Aspen Hill, Maryland. It was still dark outside, but Johnson was illuminated by the interior lights of the bus. He had a trainee with him that morning, and she immediately called 911 for help. He was conscious when fire and rescue arrived and was airlifted to Suburban Hospital. He died there several hours later. The snipers had returned once again to Aspen Hill, Montgomery County, Maryland.

Three weeks into the incident, through lengthy investigative efforts, law enforcement identified the suspects, Muhammad and Malvo. John Allen Williams (later Muhammad) was born in Louisiana in 1960. After high school, he married Carol Kaglear, had a son, and joined the National Guard. In 1985, he separated from Kaglear and joined the Army. He remarried and had three children with Mildred Green. In 1994, he left the Army, and in 1999, his second wife filed for divorce. The next year she got a restraining order against him because he had made threats against her. Soon thereafter, Muhammad fled with their three children to Antigua, where he met Malvo. Police found Muhammad and returned the children to their mother, who was now living in Maryland.

Muhammad met Malvo at a homeless shelter where they were both living. They developed a father-son relationship. In 2001, Muhammad changed his name from Williams to Muhammad and returned to the United States, bringing Malvo with him. While living in Washington State, Muhammad taught Malvo how to shoot a rifle.

They were believed to be operating a blue 1990 Chevy Caprice with New Jersey tag NDA21Z. Investigators were faced with a dilemma: Should they release the information to the media so that the public would be on the lookout for the vehicle? The concern was that the suspects could get rid of the vehicle and disappear into the shadows. Law enforcement decided to give the information to members of the media, who broadcast it over local TV and radio stations. The media announcement alerted a citizen named Whitney Donahue, who spotted the suspect vehicle on October 24, 2002, at a secluded rest area on Interstate 70 west of Frederick, Maryland. Donahue, a refrigerator repairman, was returning from some work in the Washington, DC, area to his home in Pennsylvania. He pulled into the rest area around 1:00 a.m. to break up the trip and get some sleep.

When Donahue pulled into the rest area, he observed a blue Chevy Caprice backed into a parking spot. He realized that this may be the suspect vehicle that law enforcement was searching for and located the tag number he had written down from the radio broadcast. It matched that of the sniper vehicle. The car had heavily tinted windows, so he could not see if anyone was inside. He parked in the rear of the lot, called 911, and remained on the line until the takedown occurred. Donahue was driving, of all things, a white van. MSP received the call and covertly sealed off the area.

Earlier, around 12:45 a.m., a call had come into the MCPD 911 Emergency Center from a pay phone outside the Nolte Community Center in Silver Spring. The community center is surrounded by a small wooded area. The caller claimed to be the sniper and requested police respond to this location. We figured it was either a bogus call or we were being set up for an ambush. Initially, responding SWAT units set up a perimeter and cleared parked vehicles in the area. The MSP Dauphine helicopter flew over the park area with its forward-looking infrared (FLIR), which detects heat sources, and found nothing. Our teams were preparing to enter the woods with night vision gear to clear the park. We had responded in the command vehicle to help coordinate the final search with the on-scene units.

Then, at about 1:30 a.m., we heard from the JOC that it had located the suspect vehicle at an interstate rest stop fifty miles away in rural Maryland. We were told to proceed there immediately. Minutes later, we were contacted again. The task force wanted Runk, Pierce, and me to respond to Richard Montgomery High School in Rockville, where a state police helicopter would take us to a forward staging area in Myersville. The idea was to get the team leaders there before the main tactical element to have an operational plan in place upon their arrival. Since the incident was outside of Montgomery County, FBI HRT became the lead tactical agency. FBI Team Leader Pierce did a great job of putting together the operational plan.

When we arrived at the high school, an MSP Dauphine helicopter was waiting for us on the football field. I did a quick double-check of all my gear. The co-pilot directed us to our seats and did double-checks of our harness belts. They gave us headsets for communicating with the pilot. It was a clear, crisp night with temperatures in the low fifties. The pilot informed us it would be a sixteen-minute flight. While we were en route, I looked below and saw a column of tactical vehicles proceeding "priority" north on Interstate 270 with emergency lights on.

A nineteen-man SWAT team had been assembled, five from MCPD, five from the state police, and nine from the FBI's HRT. Runk, Pierce, and I would be part of the six-man "assault element" that would include the FBI's William T. McCarthy, Paul T. Jaskot, and Neil Darnell.

Among others responding were MCPD SWAT Officer Paul Bandholz, who happened to be riding with FBI HRT operator Bill McCarthy. Paul described McCarthy as a great dude and a top-notch operator. They were at the McDonald's at New Hampshire Avenue and Route 29 in Silver Spring eating french fries when the lookout for the suspect vehicle was broadcast on the news. Seconds later, he got a call from the command post that the suspect vehicle had been spotted and they were to respond priority to the Myersville forward staging area. He drove his Ford Crown Vic "code three" with lights and siren, traveling at 100-plus mph most the trip. When they arrived, they were briefed. Bandholz was assigned to the perimeter element and McCarthy to the six-man assault team. Bandholz did a final check of his gear, grabbed some extra loaded magazines for his MP5 submachine gun, and prepared to deploy.

The helicopter landed in Myersville on a concrete roadway adjacent to a Burger King lot. The co-pilot exited the aircraft, opened the door for us, and pointed to a waiting MSP cruiser that transported us to the other side of the road to a McDonald's lot that was the staging area. Gary Bald of the FBI was the special agent in charge.

The suspect vehicle was backed in and parked along a wood line in a defensive posture. This enabled the occupants of the Caprice to see all the vehicles that entered the rest stop from the on-ramp or exited via the off-ramp. Runk, as a state trooper, had visited the rest stop many times and knew it well. He drew up a diagram of the layout of the rest stop on a pad of paper.

Pierce, the assault team leader, figured that if the suspects were in the car, they were probably resting, one in the front driver's seat and one in the back.

The plan was to deploy sniper teams into the wood line first and clear the woods with thermals and night vision gear. A concern was that if the suspects were not in the vehicle, they could be in the woods behind it. This would clear a path to the vehicle for the assault team.

The sniper teams would then be strategically placed on-line to cover the approach of the assault team. In addition, a perimeter team was deployed on-line in a wooded area to the left flank of the sniper teams to cover the ramp back to the interstate highway from the rest stop. The sniper teams and perimeter teams in combination formed a tactical "L," each with overlapping, interlocking designated fields of fire. The entire parking lot and its buildings were covered. State police had positioned a tractor trailer covertly out of sight of the suspect vehicle to block the ramp back to the interstate. The state police had shut down the interstate in both directions around the rest stop to keep all vehicle traffic out of the area. They provided the explanation that there was an accident on the interstate so as not to draw media attention to the rest stop.

The assault team would approach the vehicle from behind and from the darkness of the wooded area. The four FBI HRT operators would handle the breach and extraction of anyone inside the vehicle. Two FBI HRT operators would breach and extract from the left side on the front driver's door, and two would breach and extract from the right side on the rear passenger door. I would post on the trunk's left side as a designated shooter, supporting the FBI HRT element's left side. Runk posted on the trunk's right side, supporting the HRT element's right side as a designated shooter.

Before we left for the rest area, the assault team did a dry run on a state police car since we were a mix-and-match team, while Pierce finalized the details of the operation with Gary Bald. Pierce cautioned us not to turn on the powerful illumination lights attached to our weapons until the breaching started. We did not want to compromise our approach.

HRT operators Matt R. Lotspeich and John W. Landman briefed the sniper and perimeter teams on their assignments. Lotspeich and Landman joined the following personnel assigned to the sniper teams: FBI HRT operators Robert Hayes Parton, Thomas G. Rowan, and Keith D. Evans; MSP SWAT Troopers Sean Morris and Corporal Dale Carnegie; and MCPD SWAT Officers Dan Maddox and Dave Thomas.

The perimeter element consisted of Montgomery County SWAT Officers Paul Bandholz and John McGaha and State Police SWAT

Troopers Steve Sam and Corporal Robert McAfee. The members of the perimeter element were told that if by chance the car broke away from the vehicle assault team, they were not to let it reach the highway under any circumstance.

The task force contacted the Federal Aviation Administration (FAA) to have the airspace around the rest stop "restricted" to keep out potential press helicopters that could compromise the operation.

After our practice run, MSP cars with their lights out drove the nineteen-man tactical element to the lower entrance of the rest stop well out of sight of the suspect vehicle.

We quietly exited the vehicles. Runk and Pierce did a recon up the ramp, staying low and in the shadows until they could see the positioning of the Caprice in the bright lights of the rest stop. They could not determine if anyone was in the vehicle. Simultaneously, the sniper teams cleared the wood line and set up in their positions, and the perimeter team deployed. It was now 3 a.m.

When the sniper and perimeter teams were in place, FBI HRT Special Agent Lotspeich responded to our location and gave us a quick brief. He said the sniper teams had confirmed the tag number was that belonging to the suspect vehicle. The sniper teams had detected no movement in the vehicle. There were two rows of parking places, and the vehicle was backed in on the nearest east row, slightly favoring the left side of the lot. HRT Team Leader Pierce went over the assault plan one last time. Lotspeich then led our assault team through the woods past the sniper teams and to the car. We moved up the berm and into the woods in staggered file formation following Lotspeich. I was the last man in the column. It was very dark, and I watched where each man stepped in front of me taking the same position as we moved. My steps were slow and deliberate. We were all in black tactical uniforms, wore heavy body armor and helmets, and were heavily armed. FBI HRT and Runk, from the state police SWAT Team, were all armed with .223-caliber rifles or carbines. I was armed with a Heckler and Koch 9mm MP5A3 submachine gun. All of our weapons were equipped with white-light illumination systems.

After moving about seventy yards, we turned left (west), and I could see the parking lot lights. We were about eighty yards away from the edge of the east row where the vehicle was parked. We were now on final approach coming up behind the vehicle, the trunk facing us. We were about fifty yards from the target vehicle, and the woods started to thin. The point man did a good job of keeping what trees remained between us and the vehicle as we continued to close. We stopped and took a position of cover behind two big oak trees just at the edge of the woods.

Here we split and stacked into our two elements, the left- and right-side elements. Now we were about twenty yards from the rear of the suspect vehicle. Beyond, the woods thinned to almost nothing. This was our last position of cover and concealment. Once we left the wood line, we would be exposed and be illuminated by the bright lights at the rest stop. Since the Caprice had heavily tinted windows, we still could not see if anyone was inside. It would take only a few seconds to rush the car. The worst case would be if the vehicle went "mobile." The keys would probably be in the ignition. We were confident we could reach the vehicle before they could react.

Pierce held up three fingers and silently counted down three, two, one. We rushed the vehicle. Pierce and Jaskot breached the driver's side door and shouted, "FBI. Hands up." At the sound of breaching glass, Runk and I, who were posted on the trunk as designated shooters, activated our light systems and could clearly see inside the vehicle. Malvo, who was the lookout, had fallen asleep in the driver's seat. He was quickly extracted by Jaskot and Pierce out the driver's door. Muhammad suddenly sat up directly in front of me in the back seat and raised his hands. Runk and I covered him as he slid across the back seat following the commands of HRT operators McCarthy and Darnell. They extracted him out of the right rear passenger side of the vehicle, and he was immediately cuffed.

With both suspects secure, I took three steps back to get a better angle and covered the locked trunk. I called to Runk to get the keys from the ignition, which he did quickly and returned. He dropped to one knee, staying low, inserted the key, and prepared to unlock the trunk. I gave a nod to Runk, who unlocked the trunk and pushed it open. One of the HRT operators and I covered the trunk while Runk carefully opened it. "Clear!" called the FBI operator. "Clear!" I called out.

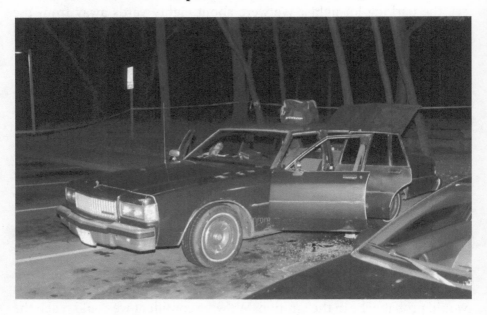

Aftermath of the vehicle assault that resulted in the capture of Malvo and Muhammad
(Courtesy of law enforcement sources)

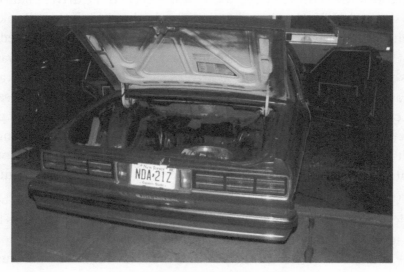

Sniper hide in the trunk of the Caprice
(Courtesy of law enforcement sources)

It was quick and decisive. From the moment we swiftly broke from the wood line, the breach and extraction of both suspects and cleared the trunk, took approximately 45 seconds.

I was looking at the trunk and noticed a small lateral, oblong cut just above the license plate. The car was pretty beat up with minor damage, and the cut appeared to be consistent with the overall appearance of the Caprice. It almost looked like someone had tried to break into the trunk. I didn't recognize it for what it was. FBI HRT operator Landman, standing next to me, pointed out that there was a dark colored sock in the hole to camouflage its appearance. It was a shooting port, or a sniper hide in the vehicle's trunk, from which the suspects shot victims.

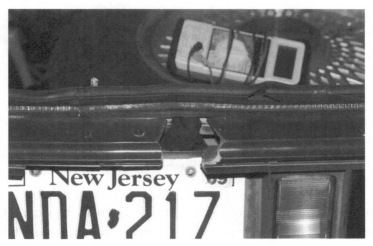

Shooting port in the trunk of the Caprice
(Courtesy of law enforcement sources)

I was told later that the idea was copied from the Irish Republican Army (IRA). Research showed the IRA historically used vehicle sniper hides with some success in Northern Ireland. The sniper teams, perimeter team, and other law enforcement agencies under the direction of HRT operators Lotspeich and Landman completed a perimeter sweep of the entire rest stop.

We turned the suspects over to the state police and the FBI. Pierce, the FBI HRT leader, commented that there was something unusual about the appearance of the back seat. After the tactical units had left, evidence technicians searched the vehicle. Behind the back-seat cushion, they found a Bushmaster XM15 E2S rifle, the bipod folded under the barrel. The rifle had a loaded magazine in it and a live round in the chamber. The rifle was held in place by a bungee cord system. A .223-caliber round was found in the parking lot as well.

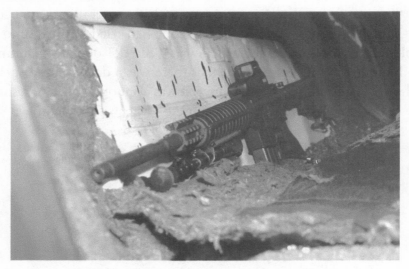

Bushmaster XM15 E2S, .223-caliber rifle fastened with
bungee cord inside the back-seat cushion
(Courtesy of law enforcement sources)

I now began to understand as we drove back to Montgomery County how the hundreds of vehicle stops we had made, the numerous buildings we had searched, the wood lines we had cleared, and all the other events we had responded to were all rehearsals for the final operation. Over the last three weeks, tactical officers from three different agencies were not riding together; they were learning together. We were communicating, playing off each other, and making our movements second nature to one another. The ability to work together greatly contributed to the success of the final operation. I took away many lessons learned from this incident.

All the overnight tactical teams in the county returned to the MCPD Academy for the morning shift change. Pierce, the FBI HRT team leader, briefed the morning tactical teams.

Afterward, I saw Pierce in the hallway at the academy and thanked him for taking members of the MCPD and MSP SWAT teams along. FBI HRT had sufficient numbers still in the county, and they could have handled the operation themselves. It was very personal for the MCPD. Our county had suffered the most casualties: Six of the ten killed in the DC region were in Montgomery County. One of those killed, Sonny Buchanan, was the son of a retired MCPD officer. The snipers also affected our ability to bury one of our own officers, Bill Faust, in peace at the Gate of Heaven Cemetery. The MSP had been at our side since Day One. Pierce and the FBI understood this. Pierce said: "We started as a team and finished as a team." This incident reinforced the strong bond that already existed among our SWAT team, the FBI HRT, and MSP SWAT.

Many years later, I met the hero of the day: Whitney Donahue, the repairman who had spotted the suspect vehicle and called police. He described the comical exchange with his wife when he arrived home at 5:30 a.m. She was not happy to be disturbed at that hour.

"There is something I need to tell you," he told her.

His wife said: "This better be good!"

Malvo and Muhammad were responsible for thirteen shootings in the Washington metropolitan region. They were ultimately linked to twenty-three shootings across the country. Both were tried and convicted of murder in Virginia. Muhammad was sentenced to death and executed by lethal injection on November 10, 2009.

Malvo was sentenced to six consecutive life sentences without the possibility of parole. In 2017, Malvo's conviction to a life sentence without parole was overturned on appeal in Virginia. The U.S. Supreme Court had ruled in *Miller v. Alabama* in 2012 that mandatory life sentences for juveniles were unconstitutional. The U.S. Supreme Court is set to review the case with respect to Malvo's sentencing and determine if the sentence stands.

This incident led to some much-needed equipment changes on our SWAT team. Our Heckler and Koch MP5A3 9mm submachine guns had an effective firing range of 100 to 200 yards. In contrast, the Bushmaster XM15 E2S .223-caliber rifle the snipers were using had an effective range of 500 to 600 yards.

We were outgunned because the snipers had a weapon with greater effective distance, and their weapon was capable of penetrating some levels of body armor. We replaced our MP5s with Colt .223-caliber carbines.

Remembering this incident only strengthened my resolve to remain in SWAT and determine what was wrong with me physically. I made an appointment with my primary physician, who referred me to John Wallmark, MD, oncology/hematology.

On August 11, 2010, I had my first consultation with Dr. Wallmark. We recognized each other because we trained at the same gym. Early on, it was determined that I had hereditary hemochromatosis, a disorder in which there is too much iron (ferritin) in the blood. This potentially could be the cause of my symptoms. I had a phlebotomy every two months, which eventually normalized the ferritin levels. However, my condition did not improve. I was getting worse, and it was becoming much more difficult to run. The shortness of breath was much more pervasive, I experienced chest discomfort, and I started to get swelling in the lower extremities.

Thereafter, I went through a vast array of specialists and testing, including chest X-ray, right upper quadrant sonogram, pulmonary function test, colonoscopy, and other tests. I began to recount other significant incidents that I had been involved in during my time in SWAT. Remembering these incidents further strengthened my resolve to stay in the unit.

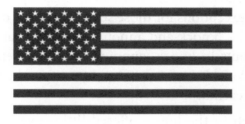

2. Hells Angels Raid

Zapped

On July 24, 2003, we assisted the ATF with a series of simultaneous raids in six states on the East Coast against the Hells Angels Motorcycle Club. The Hells Angels club had more than 2,000 members worldwide at the time, and some local chapters had a history of criminal activity.

The group had expanded into Calvert County, Maryland, about seven months earlier, according to investigators. The target location for our SWAT team was a two-level single-family home in Calvert County. We believed it was occupied by the club's vice president, Lewis J. Hall (white male, thirty-three years old), and his wife. In May of 2002, a member of a rival motorcycle club, the Pagans, had shot and wounded Hall outside a bar in Anne Arundel County. The shooter was arrested and eventually pleaded guilty to reckless endangerment. It was believed there were other individuals at the residence who may include an unidentified "hit man" from New York.

The raids targeted illegal gun and drug activity being conducted by the Hells Angels. In the early morning hours of July 24, we executed a federal "no-knock" search warrant. A no-knock warrant allows law enforcement to enter a residence without knocking at the front door or other entry point to alert those individuals inside prior to entry. Judges grant no-knock exceptions for those search warrants deemed to be high risk. In contrast, a "knock and announce" search warrant requires law enforcement agents to knock, announce their presence, and give the occupants a reasonable amount of time to respond and open the door before we can breach it.

The approach to the house offered little cover and concealment. We would use a "bail" in front of the target address. During a bail, the raid van pulls up in front of the target residence, SWAT officers exit the vehicle as quickly as possible, and the team moves toward the location in a brisk, controlled fashion. The doors to the raid van are slightly open prior to arriving to make as little noise as possible while the team exits. We quickly exited the van as we arrived and moved toward the front door, our primary entry point. The tactical medics quietly shut the van doors.

I had done the recon on the location and led the team to the front door. The door was an inward-opening wood door with a wood frame and a deadbolt lock mechanism. Two officers carried the 90-pound battering ram to the door while other officers had designated coverages on the two-level, single-family home as we approached. Quietly, I placed tape over the peephole, and I turned the knob to the door and gave a thumbs-down, indicating a locked door. The battering ram team moved into position, swung the ram, and breached the door with one hit. The door flew open, officers immediately shouted "Police search warrant" as we entered moving to our assigned areas. Large emblems clearly displayed the word "Police" on the front and back of our body armor, all standard protocol for MCPD SWAT search warrant entries.

I was Number 2 through the door after the shield man, who carried the ballistic shield. Upon entry, I immediately noticed the house was very open with high ceilings, and there were ground-level bedrooms running alongside the left interior of the house. There also appeared to be a loft area on the second level that looked out over Level 1 of the house. With another officer, I entered and cleared a bedroom immediately to my left. This was designated Bedroom 1. The bedroom was vacant, and as I exited the bedroom, I could hear some commotion coming from Bedroom 2, a second bedroom to the left beyond Bedroom 1. The first officer to enter Bedroom 2 was Reinold Winterhalter, who went to the right. Directly behind him, John McGaha went left. When McGaha entered the room, there was a bed to the left, and he proceeded to the foot of the bed. He immediately saw two bodies in the bed. Moving to the left, he was now focused on the individual on the left side of the bed as that subject was jumping out from under the covers. McGaha leveled his shotgun at that subject and began yelling, "Police search warrant. Get on the ground." McGaha recalled training he had received at the Federal Law Enforcement Training Center in Georgia in which an instructor taught a class on outlaw motorcycle clubs and how ruthless and vicious they were.

Officer McGaha could now see the subject was Hall, the vice president identified in the pre-raid brief. Hall was in a seated position with his feet on the floor. McGaha continued to tell him to get on the floor. He said it almost appeared to be in slow motion. Hall looked to his left and then turned his head to the right as both Hall's and McGaha's eyes focused on an unholstered handgun on a nightstand just a foot away from Hall's right hand. The subject then looked back at McGaha as if he was assessing his options. Hall suddenly stood up and charged McGaha without the handgun. McGaha came off target and gave a quick butt stroke with the shotgun to the advancing Hall in an effort to create distance. McGaha struck the left shoulder hard, but the subject seemed unfazed, continued to advance, and grabbed hold of the shotgun.

What McGaha did not know at the time was that the subject was on PCP (Phencyclidine), a drug used for its mind-altering effects. It can make a person aggressive and extremely violent. It reduces the pain threshold, making an individual oblivious to pain, and it is thought to make a person stronger. It can cause hallucinations and bizarre psychotic behavior.

McGaha and Hall were mirror images facing each other, both of them with hands on the shotgun and it appeared the suspect with a crazed look was gaining control. This was the moment I entered the bedroom and observed the struggle. I acquired Hall in the sights of my MP5 submachine gun and yelled to McGaha, "I'm going to shoot him," to warn McGaha of the potential shot, and hoping the words bring compliance from Hall. They did not. Knowing the shot was imminent, McGaha thrust his gun forward to break it free and push Hall away. McGaha's quick thrust and pull let him regain full control of the shotgun. He immediately went at Hall again, striking him hard and forcing him to the ground. I rushed over and jumped on top of Hall in an attempt to handcuff him. It was like a riding a wild buffalo.

Numerous other SWAT officers responded to the room. Officers called for TASERs "up" in an effort to get the subject to comply. The TASER is a non-lethal gun that fires two darts intended to puncture the skin and remain attached to the target. The darts are connected to the main unit by a thin, insulated copper wire designed to deliver an electric shock. While the electric shock is being administered, it causes temporary neuromuscular incapacitation of the subject. That shock often allows law enforcement to handcuff a combative individual.

Several officers responded with TASERs. Unfortunately, because I was intertwined and wrestling with the subject, I also received the TASER strikes. I am not sure if a dart attached to me or it was my positioning. Each time a TASER delivered an electric shock to the suspect, I too got zapped. I tried to say, "You got me," but I could never get the full sentence out, only "you got." Guys later said they thought I was saying "oh god," but I could never finish the sentence. This went on for an extended period until they finally handcuffed the subject. Multiple TASERs were used to gain compliance from the subject, and McGaha said he wasn't sure how many TASERs were involved or how many times the subject was TASED, but it was by far the most he had ever seen. I rolled off the subject, and I felt like a burned french fry.

We located four subjects: Hall, his wife, and two others. Maryland SWAT teams executed three other raids that morning. ATF reported the Maryland raids produced more than twenty guns and substantial amounts of drugs. Federal officials also reported arresting thirty members of the Warlocks Motorcycle Club on drug and gun charges as a result of the multi-state East Coast raids.

The team loaded back into the raid van for the long ride back to Montgomery County. Guys laughed and joked about the fact that I had been TASED so many times. I was sitting on one of the bench seats in the back of the raid van when, about ten minutes into the drive back, I suddenly felt a chill run through me, and my body shook for about three seconds. It was crazy; it was like an electric shock went through me. Steve Browne looked at me perplexed and asked me, "What just happened?" I explained, and he declared to the team, "It must be residual TASER shock!" Everyone laughed. On the ride home, several times guys started shaking, and a teammate asked, "Are you okay?" "Must be residual TASER shock" was the response. We all laughed. The best part of the job by far is the joking and camaraderie with teammates.

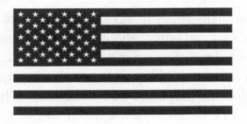

3. Serial Bank Robbers

Wet Willy

S tarting in January of 2004, the Washington metropolitan region began experiencing what the press described as a series of commando-style serial bank robberies. Multiple suspects wearing body armor and masks entered the banks with assault rifles and handguns. They quickly seized control of the banks and fired shots into the ceiling on two occasions.

In the first bank robbery, on January 22, 2004, four suspects fled with $144,000 from the Bank of America branch on Blair Road in Silver Spring, Maryland (Montgomery County). Three more holdups would take place in Washington, DC, and two in Prince George's County, Maryland. The six bank robberies yielded $360,000 in cash.

During a robbery of a Chevy Chase Bank in Prince George's County, three suspects opened fire at responding police, firing thirty rounds. One Prince George's County Police cruiser took twenty-two hits from an AK-47. Fortunately, no officers were hit.

One of the bank robberies—a holdup at a Sun Trust Bank on Connecticut Avenue NW in Washington, DC—was filmed by a WTTG-

TV (Channel 5) news crew that was in the area on assignment.

John Walsh featured the group on *America's Most Wanted,* based on the violent nature and brazen tactics of the gang. The WTTG video footage of the robbery was played on *America's Most Wanted* and described by Walsh with these words, "You are about to see some of the most dramatic pieces of video we have ever shown." The WTTG cameraman who filmed it said, "I was so focused when I saw that guy walk up to that corner with that gun. That gun was nasty looking. He had his black mask on. Whoa!" The cameraman continued to film as two other masked, heavily armed individuals ran from the bank, jumped into a van, and fled at a high rate of speed. The gang's bold tactics put the public on edge.

During each robbery, the suspects fled the scene in a stolen vehicle. They parked a second vehicle nearby. They would burn the first vehicle and then leave the area in the second vehicle.

The FBI, the U.S. Marshals Service, and local law enforcement started to gather intelligence on the group in an attempt to locate and apprehend them.

Ultimately, nine individuals would be identified, apprehended, and charged. The leader, Miquel Morrow, was also wanted on two homicide warrants.

On July 3, 2004, we had just completed an early morning raid for the Rockville City Police Department. At that time, our two SWAT supervisors were out of town. Common practice was to put the senior SWAT officer in charge of the team in the absence of the supervisors. That day, the responsibility was mine; I became the acting team leader.

After our raid, I received a call from the U.S. Marshals Service advising that they had located the suspects in the serial bank robberies. The suspects were believed to be occupying a third-floor apartment in Silver Spring, Maryland, at 14132 Grand Pre Road, #33.

The Marshals Service was asking for our assistance in the arrest of the suspects. The marshals had arrest warrants and a no-knock search warrant for the residence. We met with the marshals at a covert staging location in proximity to the target location.

While we were developing our operational plan, I sent one of our MCPD SWAT officers to do a recon. The officer who does the recon is called "security," and it is his responsibility to gather a vast quantity of information about the target location.

He will gather information about the door systems—specifically, door composition (metal, fiberglass, wood, glass, other), frame (metal, wood, unknown), locking mechanisms (knob, deadbolt, rim, chain, other), swing of the door (right to left, left to right), inward or reverse opening. Is there a peephole? If it is not an apartment, is there a storm door?

Based on intelligence gathered, we would determine a point or multiple points of entry and method of breach. Breaches fall into five categories: manual (unlocked door), mechanical (battering ram, a hydraulic device called a rabbit tool, halogen tool), ballistic (shotgun frangible round that disintegrates into tiny particles on impact), explosive (charge), and thermal (torch).

The security officer will also develop a floor plan, which we can often achieve by searching our raid database. For every raid we have ever done, we have completed and filed a floor plan or layout in our database, which contains thousands of floor plans. If nothing is in our database, we then look at similar structures in the neighborhood or examine tax records that designate square footage of a structure, number of bedrooms, etc. We use satellite photos as well. These are just some of the methods we use to obtain a layout of the target location quickly.

The security officer will gather intel on our approach and determine if we should do a bail or concealed approach. Ideally, we want a concealed approach that keeps us undetected until we reach our entry points. The security officer is also looking for motion sensors, cameras, or dogs—anything that may compromise our approach or obstacles that we have to traverse. The security officer drives the raid van to the target location because he has been to the neighborhood and seen the residence. He knows the route best and where to park, whether it be a bail or stealth approach. He is the most familiar with the approach, the neighborhood, and the residence.

The security officer returned with the following intel: We would execute a concealed deployment. We could park our raid vans out of sight of the target apartment but close by. The apartment building had an open stairwell with four apartments on each floor. The target apartment was one of two apartments on the third floor, top right. All of the target apartment's windows faced the building's rear with no view of the building's front or the entrance to the stairwell. This meant that if the stairwell was clear, we could get to the target apartment's front door undetected. The door system had a Class-2 metal door, a deadbolt and chain locking mechanism, and a metal frame. It was an inward-opening door that swung from left to right.

I suggested we use explosives to facilitate a quick breach and entry. I also suggested deploying two sniper teams and two gas teams in the event it turned into a barricade. The marshals agreed.

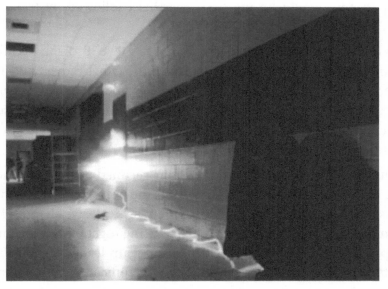

Explosive breach training
(Courtesy of MCPD)

The target apartment's door system was ideally suited for a water impulse charge. Explosive breaching is a calculated science, designed to use the minimum amount of explosive to guarantee a positive breach. It does not create a huge explosion and does not send debris and fragmentation everywhere. It is quite the opposite because one must remember one of its primary uses is in hostage-rescue incidents, where avoiding injury to the hostages is paramount. It involves surgical precision.

Anytime we do an explosive breach in an apartment stairwell, a concern we have is for the safety of the occupants of the other apartments on that floor. As we place the explosive charge on the target door, simultaneously other SWAT officers tie off with rope the other doors on that landing. This prevents occupants of the other apartments from opening their doors during the breach.

The marshals had eight tactical operators whom we would integrate into our entry team. We decided that MCPD SWAT would deploy the two sniper teams and the gas teams. We also decided that MCPD SWAT would handle the explosive breach. The first eight entry personnel into the apartment would be the U. S. marshals, followed by five MCPD SWAT officers in support.

While prepping the explosive charge, Steve Browne recalls me handing him the charge and saying to him, "Don't move," and then I walked away to get some equipment. He would later become one of our explosive breachers. His thoughts were comical as he recalled that moment. He was thinking, "This guy just handed me a bomb and said, 'Don't move,' and then left."

Our SWAT team at that time had four certified explosive breachers. Three of them were out of town, and I was the only one left. Time was of the essence. It was my responsibility to prep the explosive charge, place it, and initiate it. I was going to need help putting together the operational lineup and running the team. I turned the team leader responsibilities over to Dave Thomas, the next senior SWAT officer. A very competent and skilled operator, he quickly put together an integrated entry team of U.S. marshals and MCPD SWAT.

The team was briefed on assignments. Our sniper teams and gas teams deployed, and once they were in position, we loaded the U.S. marshals and MCPD SWAT into our two raid vans. Everyone takes a predetermined seat in the van based on assignment. This makes for a speedy, efficient exit from the van. It was a short five-minute drive to the apartment complex.

We were on our way, and I was sitting in the back of the raid van holding the explosive charge and firing device with both hands. We were reviewing our assignments, and Paul Bandholz was sitting next to me. I remembered I did not have ear protection on, critical protection from the noise of an explosive breach. I exclaimed, "I need ears for my ears!" In classic Bandholz style, he calmly placed his index finger in his mouth and then inserted it into my ear, giving me the perfect "wet willy." I was appalled, and he said the expression on my face was priceless. It was epic; the team burst out into laughter and inserted a pair of soft ear protection into my ears.

We parked and quietly exited the vans, gently shutting the doors, and did a concealed deployment to the building. The stairwell was clear as we approached, and we were able to reach the third-floor landing undetected. The security officer led us to the target door. Upon reaching it, he placed a piece of duct tape over the peephole so anyone inside the apartment would see nothing through the peephole. The security officer cautiously and gently turned the doorknob and pushed the door to determine if it was unlocked. It was locked, and he gave a thumbs-down, the hand signal to indicate the door was locked and that a breach was necessary to achieve entry.

Seeing the thumbs-down sign, the team prepared for the breach. I moved to the target door and placed the water impulse charge about three inches to the doorknob's right. I had already pulled the two-sided tape for adhesion because I did not want to make any noise in front of the door. The security officer covered the door with his firearm as I placed the charge. Simultaneously, two other MCPD SWAT officers tied off the other three apartments on the third-floor landing.

We all completed our assignments at about the same time and retreated down to the stairs leading up to the landing. The entire entry team was positioned here, crouched and stacked in a predetermined order. The stairs allowed us to be lower than the explosive charge itself.

This was important because it shielded the team from the blast and also protected the team from the overpressure associated with any explosion. The overpressure would simply pass over the top of us and vent out the open stairwell into the parking lot. We all had eye protection and ear protection for safety.

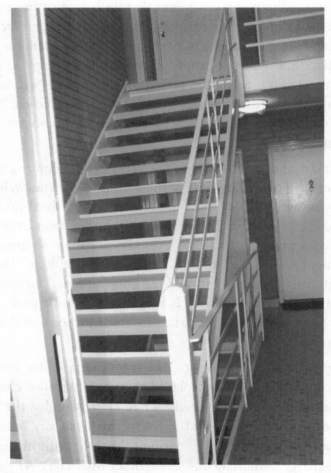

Serial bank robbers: The stairwell the team stacked on during the explosive breach, staying lower than the target door at top right
(Courtesy of MCPD)

I positioned myself as the Number 3 man in the stack. From here I could see the target door and all the other doors on the landing. I stayed to the far right on the stairs while the rest of the team favored the far left side of the stairs. This would provide a clear and unobstructed path for the team to move quickly to the door once we initiated the charge. I would stay out of their way as the team passed and would fall in as the last man to the door after the blast.

We were ready. I squeezed the right shoulder of the Number 2 man in front of me with my right hand. He squeezed the shoulder of the Number 1. Both gave me thumbs-up. I looked behind me down the stairs, and the last man in the stack gave me a thumbs-up, indicating that the rest of the team was ready. I took one last glance at the target door to ensure the charge was still secured to the door and a quick glance at the other three apartments on the landing to make sure they were still tied off. All appeared good, so I initiated the charge with my firing device. The explosion was amplified in the narrow stairwell and echoed into the parking lot. The team moved quickly to the door. It was a positive breach, and we achieved entry. The U.S. marshals, supported by MCPD SWAT, moved swiftly through the apartment, clearing the living room, kitchen, bath, and bedrooms. They secured the occupants before the suspects could react.

We took three suspects into custody, including the leader, Miquel Morrow. We also recovered firearms and body armor. U.S. marshals escorted the suspects out of the apartment, transported them, and served arrest warrants.

I examined the front door, conducting in the breaching world what is called a post-blast analysis. The charge had worked perfectly. There was a twelve-inch vertical bend in the metal door, shrinking the door smaller than the frame that it sits in. Water cannot be compressed, and the force from the water impulse charge pushed the door open, dislodging the lock mechanisms. There was no fragmentation of the door.

Immediately to the left as we entered was a black sofa backed along the wall with a white landline phone sitting on its right arm. About six feet slightly to the right sitting across from it was a matching black recliner. Nestled between these items was a brown wooden coffee table with a beer on it. The apartment was cluttered and dirty. One suspect was only four feet from the door when the charge detonated. He had no injuries; the phone was still sitting undisturbed on the right arm of the couch several feet from the door, and the beer bottle was upright on the coffee table four to five feet from the door. This is a prime example of how explosive breaching, when used properly, is safe for all involved.

After every raid, we conduct a debrief in the raid van as we return to the staging location. We start with the Number 1 man and continue in sequence until every SWAT officer has spoken. Each officer talks about his assignment, what he encountered, and the actions that he took. It is important to acknowledge if we made a mistake or could have been done something better. The idea is to take away lessons learned and be more prepared for the next operation.

The raid went well, but I also reminded myself that it is important for the SWAT team to remember: "Never rest on your achievements. We are only as good as our next operation."

The U.S Marshals Service and a joint local-federal task force arrested five of the remaining six suspects. The last suspect was already in police custody on unrelated charges. The final tally recovered was seven different assault rifles, including AK-47s and machine pistols, and body armor. FBI special agent Thomas Kinnally characterized the suspects as "a particularly vicious band of thieves whose intent was to steal and terrorize innocent civilians."

I learned an important lesson during this incident. I always was of the mindset that if you want something done right, you should do it yourself. Turning the team leader responsibilities over to Dave Thomas taught me a valuable lesson about delegating authority. Thomas did a better job than I would have. It made me think of something General George S. Patton once said: "Don't tell people how to do things. Tell them what to do and let them surprise you with their results."

This significant raid resulted in the arrest of a violent group of serial bank robbers. Yet the team remembers it not for its significance as a criminal incident but rather for the wet willy that Bandholz delivered.

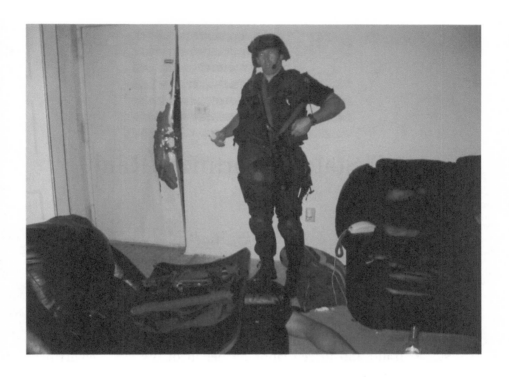

Explosive breach of door resulting in capture of three serial bank robbers
(Courtesy of MCPD)

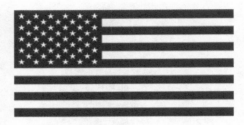

4. State Department Raid

The Unknown

On August 3, 2007, the MSP SWAT Team asked us to help serve two search warrants in Burtonsville, Maryland, for fraud and forced labor on behalf of the U.S. Department of State and the U.S. Department of Homeland Security's Immigration and Customs Enforcement.

It was rumored that the suspects had ties to a terror group in the Middle East. The residences were two single-family homes that sat across the street from each other in Burtonsville, near the end of a cul-de-sac.

We had a mix and match of personnel for the entry teams from MSP SWAT and MCPD SWAT. We did

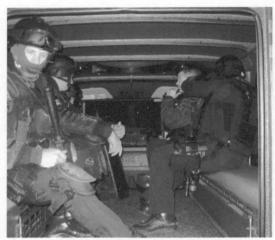

In a raid van preparing for a "hit"
(Courtesy of MCPD)

simultaneous "hits" of both structures. The approach was open and did not favor a stealth, concealed approach. We would do a bail in front of the target addresses. As raid vans approached, the doors were, as usual, already partially ajar, allowing for a quick exit from the vehicle. Teams advanced to the front doors of both locations. The tactical medics locked and secured the vehicles.

The search warrants were "knock and announce," requiring law enforcement to knock and announce their presence before entering. At each location, police knocked at the front door and loudly announced: "Police search warrant. Open the door." After waiting a reasonable amount of time with no response and observing no movement inside, team leaders gave the order to breach the doors. Ram teams breached the doors at each location with a two-man battering ram.

My assignment was a bedroom. I was moving toward the bedroom when a subject came out of the bedroom into the living room area where I was located. I ordered him down to the ground at gunpoint and secured him with handcuffs. After turning the subject over to investigators and clearing the house, I went into the kitchen, where I found a large center island filled with pictures covered by a large, clear piece of plastic or glass. One of the first pictures I saw was a male subject similar in appearance to the individual I had "taken down" in the living room. The picture appeared to have been taken in the desert, possibly the Middle East, and that person was carrying an assault rifle and dressed in headgear and militant-type attire.

I learned that a male subject in his thirties was taken into custody at the other location and that SWAT operators observed similar militant-themed pictures there as well. Officer Bill Mcquiggan, part of the entry team, remembers a board on a wall that had the addresses and keys to properties up and down the East Coast. In the basement, there was a weight room and a full-size boxing ring. There also was a walk-in safe with a monster formidable steel door. One of our primary breachers, Mcquiggan remembers that the entry team members were trying to figure out collectively how to breach it. Then an idea hit them. The suspects spent big money on the door, but it appeared they went cheap on the surrounding wall install. Mcquiggan grabbed the sledgehammer, and they pounded their way through the drywall next to the door. It was just drywall and studs, and he thought to himself, "So much for the fancy door!" Inside the vault, they found an SKS assault rifle.

We turned the subjects over to federal authorities at both locations. We returned to our raid vans wondering what this all meant, but we never heard anything more about the incident.

Many years after this incident, I spoke with MCPD District Commander Paul Liquorie, who was a supervisor in Vice and Intelligence (V&I) when the raids occurred. He provided new insight and a measure of clarity about the circumstances that led to the raids.

Special agents from the Office of Export Enforcement (OEE) at the Department of Commerce's Bureau of Industry and Security contacted the V&I Section through the FBI Baltimore Field Office's Joint Terrorism Task Force. The OEE has a unique mission in the homeland security realm and works with other law enforcement agencies to ensure that classified and restricted technologies developed in the United States are not exported to adversaries.

This case started out as a fraud case where the target of the investigation purchased two pieces of a commercially available but restricted type of construction equipment: a type of ground-penetrating radar that may have even had some nuclear material within each device to augment the devices' capabilities. The target had ordered two devices but ultimately had not paid the invoices, so the manufacturer reported this as a fraud case. Because these were restricted devices, the OEE picked up the case after learning the purchaser was from the Middle East and then brought in Montgomery County V&I and SWAT.

Liquorie explained we helped execute the federal search warrants in hopes of recovering the devices but also were seeking packing slips, invoices, etc., as evidence of the fraud. It was quickly apparent that the main target had fled and that the family was in the process of leaving the country. There was little furniture left in the house, and they had suitcases and boxes packed throughout. Investigators may have found some invoices or packaging from the equipment in question. Thirteen years have passed since the incident, so Commander Liquorie authorized the release of details of MCPD involvement in the event. He said MCPD never knew how the case concluded because we did not have a need to know, part of working in the field of homeland security and counterterrorism.

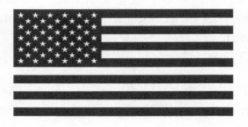

5. Officer Down

One of Our Own

In February of 2009, the Police Community Action Team (PCAT), supported by several SWAT officers, began working a saturation detail on Castle Boulevard in Silver Spring trying to suppress a wave of violent criminal activity in that area. PCAT had about eight officers, and we had three SWAT officers detailed to support them. On February 26 at 8:15 p.m., PCAT stopped two vehicles on the northbound shoulder near the 14000 block of Castle Boulevard. Kevin Reese, Andrew Ingalls, and Corporal Tom Dalbora handled the first stop. The vehicle stopped was a 1994 Pontiac Bonneville with Maryland tags. Reese detected a strong odor of marihuana coming from the vehicle. Ingalls identified the driver of the vehicle and had him step out of the vehicle and sit on the curb near the car. Corporal Dalbora had the rear passenger step out of the vehicle and sit on the curb near the rear of the vehicle. At this time, the keys were still in the ignition of the vehicle, and the car was still running.

I had just arrived backing up the officer on the second stop, which was about fifty yards behind the first stop, and exited my vehicle. Reese advised the subject in the front passenger seat, later identified as Nicholas Omar Banks, to step out of the vehicle. Banks suddenly jumped to the driver's side of the vehicle. At this time, Reese quickly ran around the front of the vehicle in an attempt to reach Banks on the driver's side and order him out of the vehicle. Banks abruptly put the vehicle in drive, stepped on the gas, and quickly accelerated with Reese directly in front of the car. The officer was struck and launched onto the hood of the car as the suspect accelerated very quickly. Perched on the hood, severely injured from the impact, he managed to draw his handgun and fired several shots through the windshield at the driver in an effort to save his own life. The car abruptly swerved to the left and crashed into a fence. The officer landed on the ground, and he was badly injured. The suspect fled on foot toward a group of townhouses on the west side of the 14000 block of Castle Boulevard.

Hearing the sound of shots, I jumped into my vehicle and raced to the first stop. I observed Reese down in the roadway and other officers attending to him. I immediately cleared the suspect vehicle making sure there were no other occupants in it. Reese had suffered severe injuries, and Corporal Dalbora advised dispatch of the situation on the police radio. I told Corporal Dalbora to take care of his down officer and that SWAT would go after the suspect. Within a minute or two, more SWAT officers were on the scene, and shortly thereafter, Darren Crandell from the Decentralized SWAT Team, who works the 3rd District where the incident occurred, arrived. Crandell was a highly motivated and skilled officer. We send our decentralized officers to a variety of tactical schools hosted by outside law enforcement agencies to gain knowledge and experience. Crandell had the uncanny ability to finish Number 1 in each school he attended. In the near future, he would be selected to the Central SWAT Team.

Sergeant Whalen, the supervisor of PCAT, arrived, and I suggested that he coordinate establishing a perimeter around the neighborhood while SWAT attempted to track the suspect with two K9 teams that had just arrived. He agreed. We deployed as two search teams. Each team had a K9 officer and dog and two SWAT officers in support. The K9 officer I was with was Bill Seidel, a former member of our Central SWAT Team. Seidel was a sharp cop; he had been a police officer in DC prior to coming to Montgomery County. He was big and strong, having played in the NFL for a year. The lookout for the suspect was for a black male wearing a gray jacket or sweatshirt with red and blue stripes. There was blood at the scene, and it was believed that the suspect had been shot. The K9 teams tracked to the rear of the nearby Briggs Chaney shopping center and then lost the track. As the track was concluding, information developed identifying the suspect as Nicholas Omar Banks, a black male, age thirty-three, 5' 11", 175 pounds who lived at 14146 Castle Boulevard, Apartment #104.

Upon learning this information, uniformed patrol officers had formed a perimeter around the building. SWAT responded, and we observed a blood trail inside the building. We tied off the apartment door at #104 with rope so that it could not be opened. It was a ground-level apartment with windows on one side only, what we referred to as the Charlie side.

I had two SWAT officers cover the door of apartment #104 from inside the stairwell. I had the third SWAT officer with support from uniform patrol officers cover the other apartments in the stairwell in case the suspect had gone to another apartment in the building. I initiated an Emergency Response Team callout to get additional SWAT officers so we could breach the door and enter to search the apartment. Upon arrival of the main SWAT element, we formed an eleven-man entry team, and five other SWAT officers deployed in the stairwell to cover other apartments. A sniper team deployed to cover the windows on the apartment's Charlie side, and a SWAT element replaced the patrol perimeter element around the apartment. Negotiators attempted to contact the occupants inside, with no response.

Investigators obtained a search warrant for the apartment, and we used an explosive water impulse charge to breach a Class-2 inward-opening metal door with a metal frame, rim lock, and deadbolt. The breach succeeded, and the entry team cleared the apartment, which we found to be vacant. In the master bedroom, we found blood-soaked clothing similar to what Nicholas Banks had been wearing. Detectives photographed the scene, collected the items inside, and placed them into evidence. With a consent search from the occupants, we cleared all other apartments in the building, except for three apartments where there was no response when SWAT knocked on the door. The suspect apparently had left the apartment during the time lapse between the search by K9 and the time it took to identify and set a perimeter around the suspect's apartment.

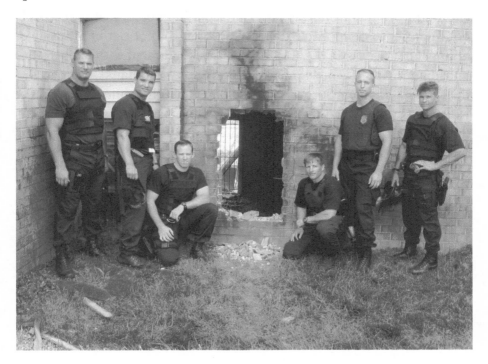

Explosive breaching element
(Courtesy of MCPD)

Information developed that the suspect may be inside an apartment at 13912 Castle Boulevard, where his girlfriend lived. Sergeant Brian Dillman (later lieutenant) led a team of SWAT officers to search and clear the apartment. Simultaneously, I led a team of officers searching with a police bloodhound that had just arrived. Bloodhounds are very effective at tracking, particularly after they have the scent of a suspect's bloodied clothes. Though the search of the girlfriend's apartment by Dillman's team was negative, she confirmed that the suspect had returned to his apartment at 14146 Castle Boulevard after the shooting, changed clothes, and left.

The bloodhound led us to a wooded area near the suspect's apartment.

We used night vision gear and conducted an extensive search. Dillman and his team searched a second wooded area based on information the girlfriend provided. The suspect was not located at either location.

It was now nearing sunrise. We decided to withdraw all the SWAT and uniform units from the neighborhood. We hoped that if all visible police presence disappeared, the suspect would come out of his place of hiding if he was still in the area. The area was saturated with plainclothes units in unmarked vehicles in an effort to apprehend Banks. Members of the Repeat Offenders Section, a group of plainclothes officers who target violent criminal offenders, were given this task. Surveillance teams monitored the area and followed up on additional leads provided by investigators. Surveillance teams worked the neighborhood extensively thereafter but were unable to locate Banks.

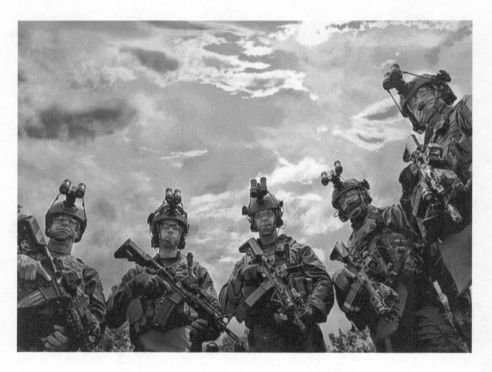

Night vision gear used in wood-line search of suspect wanted for attempted murder of a police officer; the search ended at daybreak
(Courtesy of MCPD)

A criminal history check revealed that Banks had numerous previous arrests, which may have influenced his decision to flee the police.

We transported the other two occupants of the vehicle to the Silver Spring police station, where investigators interviewed them. They weren't charged.

Reese was transported to the hospital, where he underwent surgery for multiple injuries to his left knee, right foot/leg, and both hands. Fortunately, he survived the incident.

Investigators obtained arrest warrants for Banks, initially charging him with attempted first-degree murder, attempted second-degree murder, attempted manslaughter, first-degree assault, second-degree assault, and second-degree assault on a law enforcement officer. At a later date, Banks' family members contacted law enforcement and made arrangements for his peaceful surrender to police.

Shortly after this incident in 2009, my career-long goal of becoming the SWAT commander sergeant for the MCPD came true. The previous sergeant had retired, and I had been running the team for months, filling the open position. Soon thereafter, I was joined by Sergeant Brian Dillman, the assistant commander. Aside from being a very capable leader, Dillman offered strong administrative skills that I lacked. He had a great deal of SWAT experience as well, and we worked very well together for the duration of my career.

Upon receiving the position, I met with the Central Team to share my expectations and some observations I had made as an operator with twenty-four years of SWAT experience. These guys were my best friends, and now I was going to be their supervisor. I said, "You guys are all Type A personalities. I have learned over the years watching other supervisors that I am not in charge of you; I am simply responsible for you." They all laughed, but we understood each other. Train hard, do your job, stay out of trouble, and we're good. Each person on the team did this daily, and I respected them for it. I also told them that because we were allocated time to work out to meet the required physical standards, "you are the closest thing to a professional athlete you will ever be." I also noted: "You may not make the money or receive the notoriety of a professional athlete, but you are getting paid. Being physically fit is a very important aspect of the job." I have always said the best job in this police department is being an operator as a Police Officer 3 (PO3) in SWAT. We get to work out, train in tactical skills, get the bad guys in high-profile incidents, experience adrenaline rushes, and do very little paperwork. I loved being the SWAT commander, but by far the most fun I had was as an operator.

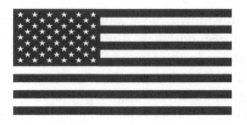

6. Discovery Suicide Bomber

Apocalypse

On September 1, 2010, just three weeks after my initial doctor's appointment, an incident occurred that would be the" finest hour" of the MCPD SWAT Team to date: The Discovery building suicide bomber hostage rescue case, which would further strengthen my resolve to stay in the unit. It had more drama than the sniper incident and far greater potential for dire consequences. Initially, it received national and international attention, but it never received the follow-up media attention that the sniper incident did, perhaps because the apex of the sniper incident lasted three weeks and involved thirteen local shootings, killing ten. The Discovery incident was over within four hours with no civilian casualties. This is the full inside story, told for the first time, on what law enforcement experts consider one of the most significant hostage rescues in law enforcement history.

It was a sunny, humid day—ninety-five degrees. I had just exited the courthouse in Rockville, Maryland. This was the final day of my divorce. My attorney said, "Jeff, you need to do something special for yourself today." We shook hands, and I walked toward my unmarked SWAT vehicle. Little did I realize that a series of events was unfolding that I would never forget.

A gunman wearing a person-borne improvised explosive device (PBIED) entered the lobby of the Discovery Communications headquarters in downtown Silver Spring. The gunman fired several shots and took three hostages. The incident was the first suicide bomber with hostages in the United States. The Discovery building is one mile north of the DC line and is in Silver Spring's central business district. Montgomery County is unique in that in most agencies, bomb technicians reside on the police side. In our jurisdiction, the bomb techs also serve as fire marshals and work under the fire-and-rescue umbrella. Montgomery County Fire and Rescue has 1,100 personnel, including an arson/explosive unit with thirteen Maryland law enforcement officers who are FBI-certified bomb techs. The unit handles about 220 suspicious-item calls per year.

The MCPD has about 1,200 officers and a full-time SWAT Team of 11 officers. The full-time SWAT Team, or Central Team, does nothing but SWAT operations. It averages 200 raids and fifteen to twenty barricades a year. The SWAT Team also does dignitary protection details, conducts and attends training, and undertakes other tactical assignments.

There is also a Decentralized SWAT (DSWAT) or part-time SWAT Team of eighteen officers who supplement the Central Team as needed. These officers are assigned to other units throughout the department and train with the Central Team at least twice a month. They also attend tactical schools each year, such as schools for snipers and explosive breaching. The Montgomery County Sheriff's Department has a six-man Special Response Team (SRT) that has completed our basic SWAT school. It is geared and outfitted the same as our DSWAT officers. They attend training twice a month with the DSWAT Team and also assist as needed. At the time of the Discovery incident, there was also one Gaithersburg City police officer who met the same criteria and supplemented us.

In 1996, SWAT Officer Rob Ulisney, a former Navy SEAL; Officer Glen Baker; and I started our SWAT Team's explosive breaching program. We attended Tactical Explosive Entry School in Mississippi and became certified explosive breachers. The school was taught by Alan Brosnan, a former commander of a New Zealand Special Air Service counterterror team. Ulisney was the only person on our SWAT Team with any previous explosives experience (from his time in the Navy), so for safety and oversight, we reached out to our bomb techs on the fire and rescue side. During our first year, anytime we trained with explosives, the bomb techs were present. What was important is that a strong relationship developed between the SWAT Team and the bomb techs.

Ulisney is one of my best friends. He brought a lot of positive change to the SWAT Team in terms of how we did a lot of things: wood-line searches, close-quarters battle, tubular assaults, and much more. He and I worked out at the gym on numerous occasions. He always elevated my game and brought out the best in me. I have always had great admiration for our elite military teams and tried to prove I was his equal in everything we did. I never was, but his presence made the rest of the team and me better.

After 9/11, several more terrorist incidents occurred across the globe.

On March 11, 2004, a series of coordinated bombings occurred in Madrid, Spain. The bombings occurred during the morning hours on the commuter train system. Al-Qaeda was the perpetrator of bombings that killed 198 and injured more than 1,400.

On July 7, 2005, a series of coordinated suicide bombings occurred at three London underground subway stations. The attacks targeted civilians in the morning hours, killing fifty-two and injuring over 700.

After the November 2008 terrorist attack in Mumbai, India, we recognized as a SWAT Team that we were not prepared for potential post-9/11 incidents of that magnitude. So we reached out to resources beyond the realm of law enforcement that we felt could best prepare us for such an event.

As a result, we developed what we call our Code Red Counter-Terror Teams. A code red incident is one that far surpasses a traditional Emergency Response Team (ERT) callout. It is most likely related to a post-9/11 incident but not necessarily so.

We took one-hundred police personnel within our department and over the course of a year trained them in various tactics and skills. Two months before the Discovery incident, we trained all one-hundred members of our Code Red Teams in several scenarios, focusing on active-shooter response and improvised explosive devices (IEDs). Just by chance, one scenario was for a suicide bomber with hostages, and the building we trained in was similar in size and design to the Discovery building. We conducted the "suicide bomber with hostages" training scenario in the building's lobby; as fate would have it, the Discovery incident occurred in the building's lobby.

We had four Code Red Teams—named gold, silver, green, and blue— designed as stand-alone teams, meaning they could perform a variety of functions independently. Each team had a SWAT component of nine officers. It also had a surveillance unit of eight plainclothes officers, a K9 team with bomb explosive-detection capability, two bomb techs, and two tactical medics.

Then New York City experienced a failed car-bombing incident on May 1, 2010. We decided that if a similar event occurred in Montgomery County, we would send a Code Red Team to the scene in addition to first responders on the street. SWAT would deploy and assume over-watch and site security duties. The plainclothes surveillance team would look for suspicious persons potentially waiting to activate secondary devices remotely on first responders. The bomb techs would assume control of the scene and device. The K9 team would start a sweep of the area for potential secondary explosive devices and call in additional dogs as needed. Tactical medics would develop contingency plans with fire and rescue in the event a device detonated.

Montgomery County has an extensive subway network and a vast commuter train system, both feeding into the nation's capital. We determined that if events occurred such as those in Madrid or London, we would send our Code Red Teams to work "post-blast" duties at affected sites.

What concerned us most was what happened in Mumbai. During the Mumbai terrorist attacks in November of 2008, two active-shooter incidents occurred simultaneously: the takeover of the Taj Mahal Hotel and the active shooters on the railway platform.

We wanted to have the ability to send two large forces as part of our initial response to meet two critical incidents occurring at once. We would combine our four Code Red Teams into two teams. Each element would provide fifty officers in addition to the first responders on the street. This would be our first action taken until we could get allied tactical teams from other agencies to support us.

The worst-case scenario from a psychological standpoint would be a school takeover. When this occurred in Beslan, Russia, on September 1, 2004, there were thirty-four terrorists. The MCPD SWAT Team with all its central and decentralized officers has only thirty-five operators. Certainly, a one-to-one ratio is insufficient for trying to take back a defensive position. However, if we combined all our Code Red Teams, we would have over one-hundred personnel plus first responders. Soon thereafter, we would receive more support from our allied tactical teams and agencies.

The fact that we had run an identical suicide bomber training scenario two months before the Discovery incident, had Code Red Teams in place, and had a strong relationship with our bomb techs provided numerous dividends as we rolled into the Discovery incident.

On September 1, 2010, James Lee entered the south lobby of the Discovery building located at One Discovery Place in Silver Spring. It is a high-rise building that occupies an entire city block in downtown Silver Spring. Silver Spring is an urbanized, unincorporated area in Montgomery County. Discovery, Inc., is the world's Number 1 non-fiction media company, reaching more than 1.5 billion subscribers in 180-plus countries. It features channels such as the Discovery Channel, The Learning Channel, Animal Planet, Discovery Kids, Discovery Travel and Living, Discovery Civilization, and Science Channel. Discovery had 1,900 staff and fifty children at a day-care center on the first floor. It provides public access through two sets of glass doors in the lobby.

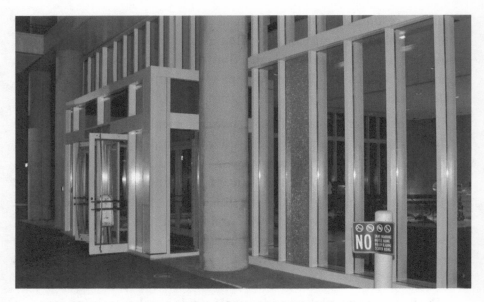

The Discovery building's south lobby entrance
(Courtesy of MCPD)

The interior of the south lobby is pristine, with polished marble floors and many displays for public viewing. Visitors enter through double glass doors. The lobby has a high ceiling and glass windows on three sides. The lobby is about 200 feet wide and eighty feet deep. It looks like a museum. At the time, there were a skeleton of a T-Rex dinosaur and cardboard cutouts of the men from the TV show *American Chopper*. Artifacts and other items were suspended from the ceiling. Three concrete pillars extending from floor to ceiling, about three feet in diameter, are evenly spaced throughout the lobby. There is a manned security kiosk in the south lobby. The security guard that day was Thomas Neil Fisher, a white male (age thirty-seven) with prior military experience. Fisher was wearing a white long-sleeve shirt and dark pants and was standing behind the desk at the security center.

James Lee, an Asian male (age forty-three), entered the lobby dressed in black from top to bottom: black pants, black short-sleeve shirt, and black baseball cap. He was pushing a wheeled cart that contained a military-style Alice pack frame and other items.

A maintenance worker, suspicious of Lee as he entered the lobby, watched as Lee approached the security desk. Lee suddenly displayed a handgun, fired three shots into the air, and took Fisher hostage. The maintenance worker immediately fled the building through the south lobby doors. Lee removed and then put on a PBIED from the cart mounted on the Alice pack and began arming the device. While he was arming his device, James Francis McNulty interrupted Lee when McNulty entered the south lobby through the lobby doors. McNulty was a white male (thirty-six) dressed in tan pants and a dark-colored, short-sleeve polo shirt. Lee pointed the handgun at McNulty and ordered him to the ground, where Lee placed him in a prone position. McNulty placed a rolling briefcase on the floor. Lee went back to arming his device when he was interrupted for a second time as Christopher Brooks Wood (white male in his thirties) entered the lobby. He was dressed in dark-colored pants and a light-colored, short-sleeve shirt. Lee also ordered Wood to assume a prone position on the floor. Lee now had three hostages. Fisher, the security guard, was a Discovery employee, as were the other two hostages. SWAT would not learn until after the incident ended that Wood and McNulty were also Discovery employees.

Numerous emergency calls began to come into the 911 center reporting a man with a gun, shots fired, and a suspect with hostages and explosives strapped to his body.

One 911 caller reported: "There is a hostage. Discovery Building. Discovery, there is someone in lobby with a gun. He came into the lobby with a revolver and told them not to leave. He looks like he has a bomb. He is in the main entrance to the building."

A responding patrol officer arriving on scene reported the following over the police radio: "He looks like he has an IED, looks like he is setting up some sort of explosive device in the lobby."

A lieutenant (car 301 call sign) responded: "I need a fast-action response team to respond right here to Georgia and Wayne and to suit up to see what we have. The station shields are on way."

The district commander issued an order: "I want every officer who is in service down here now."

MCPD Officer Ed Paden was off duty driving his marked police cruiser several blocks from the Discovery building when the emergency call went out. Paden worked in the 3rd District, the area in which the incident occurred. Paden was very familiar with the Discovery building. He had worked part-time security during its construction to supplement his income. He put on his yellow police armband used to identify off-duty officers and grabbed his Benelli shotgun.

Paden advised the dispatcher: "OD 1520 [call sign], I am in the circle with a Benelli. I am in plainclothes, gray shirt, tan pants, police badge on my left shoulder." He continued, "OD 1520 to any supervisor." He was also familiar with the south lobby that Lee had seized. Paden entered the building at a safe location via the garden and made his way to the rear of the south lobby. He knew that there were two corridors at the rear of the south lobby that granted access to the rest of the building. He picked one corridor in particular to block because he knew a security office with cameras was located there. Paden accessed the camera system and provided intelligence on the device. He also directed other responding patrol officers to block the other corridor, preventing Lee from penetrating the building any farther.

A lieutenant acknowledged him: "301 [call sign], go ahead."

Paden advised: "I am almost directly behind the suspect behind a wall. I have a visual on his apparatus. I am losing battery on my portable. If you come in via the garden area, a security officer will let you in who can walk you to me." The garden area was an open space outside the west side of the building that Lee could not see

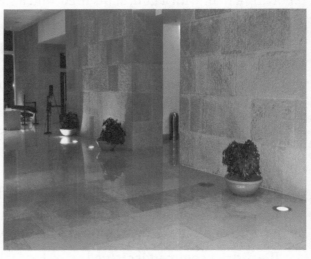

The back of the Discovery building's main lobby
(Courtesy of MCPD)

from the lobby.

Eric Mercurio, a DSWAT officer, came on the air and asked "9 Tango 33 [call sign], how can I get to him?"

Paden said: "OD 1520, come to the garden off the circle; you will see a stairwell door. There will be some employees flagging you down. They will walk you to the lobby or you can enter through Colesville. Either way, they will walk you to me." Colesville was a second lobby entrance on the building's north side, also out of Lee's sight.

Paden continued: "I have a visual on the suspect via the camera system. Like a mini backpack. Looks like two canisters on the outside and a propane bottle on the inside. Looks like two coffee cans surrounding the propane canister. Flashing light in his left hand, almost like a death grip. Red illuminous light, continuous flashing. Same thing on front strapped around his waist."

Paden did everything right, an outstanding job. Certainly, if there was a hero that day, it was Paden.

Unfortunately, a Discovery employee looking out a window many floors up in the Discovery building saw Paden outside in the garden area attempting to enter the building. That employee did not recognize the bright yellow police armband on Paden's left shoulder that identifies off-duty MCPD officers, so that person called the 911 emergency center and reported Paden as a second gunman, armed with a machine gun in the garden area.

I was notified of the incident very early on, before an ERT callout occurred. Sergeant Brady Clouser was working as patrol supervisor in the 3rd District as events unfolded. He was a former member of our Central SWAT Team who left when promoted to sergeant and remained active as a member of the DSWAT Team. Clouser had a vast amount of SWAT experience, including time on a SWAT team in Florida before coming to the MCPD.

He called me on my cell phone, gave me a quick brief, and said: "Jeff, start monitoring channel 3 [3rd District radio channel] and bring everything we have."

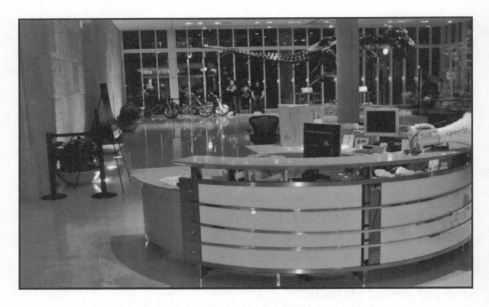

The Discovery building's main lobby and security desk
(Courtesy of MCPD)

The intel I had while en route was that a suspect with a handgun had fired shots and taken hostages in the south lobby of the Discovery building. It also appeared he had some sort of explosive device on his person. A report also identified a second suspect armed with a machine gun in the garden area. I started to think of the similarities between the terrorist attack in Mumbai and what was happening in Silver Spring. In Mumbai, active shooters overtook a significant structure—the Taj Mahal Hotel. In Silver Spring, a gunman had overtaken a significant structure—the headquarters of Discovery, the largest non-fiction media outlet in the world. In Mumbai, active shooters were on the railway platform. Two hundred yards from where Paden was misidentified as a second gunman, a subway platform feeds the Silver Spring business district.

Thinking that this might be the start of a post-9/11, multi-site attack, we activated our Code Red Teams to get as many tactical resources on site as quickly as possible to counter any other threats. Ironically, at that moment, Assistant SWAT Commander Brian Dillman was preparing to give a presentation to the visiting Mexico City chief of police on our

Code Red Counter-Terror Teams. Dillman told the visiting chief of police that a developing emergency was precipitating our Code Red Teams' first deployment, so he must leave immediately.

Dillman, a former defensive lineman on the University of Iowa football team, is massive: 6' 4" and 265 pounds. When he first came to SWAT, we lived in the same neighborhood. I had a full gym in my basement, and we often trained together. What I quickly learned was that he was an exceptional athlete, intelligent, and an excellent decision-maker in tactical situations.

His stature was reaffirmed one day when I was giving a presentation at the International Breachers Symposium attended by law enforcement and military teams. I showed a picture that included Dillman. Afterward, I was approached by members of the Norwegian Special Forces, who asked, referring to Dillman: "Who is the Viking?" I liked it, so we dubbed him "the Viking."

Dillman also has a sense of humor, which surfaced when a captain came to the SWAT office yelling, "I'm going to kick some ass!" Dillman looked around at the SWAT guys seated at their desks and calmly asked, "Captain, whose ass are you going to kick back here?" After assessing Dillman's size and demeanor, frustrated, the captain turned around and briskly walked away, continuing to yell and scream as he left. We all chuckled.

Early on at the Discovery building, an executive officer attempted to get to Paden via the garden area. Unfortunately, that officer went to the wrong door, so no one was standing by to let him in. He decided to breach the door with his handgun, so he fired several shots and gained entry. It is admirable that he was making an effort to get to Paden; however, the officer failed to notify those on scene over the police radio that he would be firing shots. This caused great confusion for a brief period because the sound of shots echoed in the area where reports had identified Paden as a second gunman. Soon thereafter, the officer acknowledged he had fired the shots. The shots could be heard from the day care center and caused concern among the employees. Fortunately, we soon determined that the Discovery employee had mistakenly identified Paden as a second gunman.

Mercurio arrived and entered the Colesville side, where a security officer met him. Mercurio directed her to stand by and keep the door open for responding SWAT units. Another security officer led Mercurio to the south lobby, where Paden was in the security office. Mercurio observed the surveillance cameras while Paden covered the corridor with his Benelli. Mercurio recalls he could clearly see three hostages and easily identify the suspect based on the fact that he was wearing what appeared to be some sort of makeshift backpack with multiple canisters of an unknown substance. The backpack was connected to a device in Lee's hand. Mercurio noticed that Lee would not loosen his grip without covering it with the other hand. It appeared the device was "release initiated," meaning it would detonate when he released his grip on it. Though Lee appeared agitated, the hostages were compliant.

Responding patrol officers and DSWAT units on scene immediately isolated Lee in the lobby. Clouser joined Mercurio in the security office. Mercurio recalls that Clouser quickly took command. He was relieved to have Clouser take charge because he knew that Clouser had been a member of the Central SWAT Team and was a capable leader. Clouser coordinated the response of responding SWAT officers and ensured that the two corridors that led off the rear of the south lobby were blocked and that the suspect was contained.

The National Capital Region, or DC area, uses a sectoring/target coding standard for law enforcement and tactical teams in the region. It uses phonetic designators to denote the sides, exposures, and interior quadrants of the building. Alpha is the building's front (street address) side. Continuing clockwise from Alpha are Bravo, Charlie, and Delta. So the left side of the building was Bravo, the rear was Charlie, and the right side Delta (see Table 1 below).

The lobby area that Lee occupied was rectangular with four distinct sides. The Alpha (street address) side faced east toward Georgia Avenue. Continuing clockwise, the double lobby doors through which Lee had entered the lobby were the Bravo side (south), left of the double doors was the Charlie side (west), and the backside of the lobby was the Delta side (north). In the lobby's backside (Delta), two corridors granted access to the rest of the building. In a stealth and covert manner, the initial responding units blocked the two corridors out of Lee's sight. The initial responding units, blocking the two corridors, formed two Immediate Action Teams (IATs)—officers prepared to prevent immediate loss of life. A perimeter of patrol officers also covered the outside of the south lobby.

Table 1. National Capital Region Designations and Positioning of Our Tactical Elements and Other Units

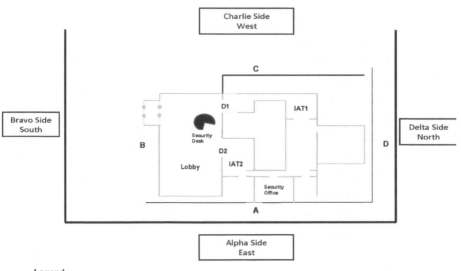

Legend

A— Alpha side of building, front of building, facing Georgia Avenue

B— Bravo side to building, double lobby doors through which suspect James Lee entered

C— Charlie side of building

D— Delta side of building, rear lobby where IATs 1 &2 staged out of suspect's sight behind a wall

- Staged distance from IAT 1 to target: ~50 feet
- Staged distance from IAT 2 to target: ~60 feet

- **IAT 1**—Became Delta 1 Assault Team when we replaced uniformed officers with SWAT officers
- **IAT 2**—Became Delta 2 Assault Team when we replaced uniformed officers with SWAT officers

- Security—Location of camera system in security office

Our SWAT tactical medics carry portable radiological detection devices to detect and measure external or ambient ionizing radiation fields. The tactical medics, positioned in support of the two SWAT Assault Teams, had no indication of radiation coming from the device.

We didn't know what the mechanism was, so we hoped this eliminated the possibility of a radiological dirty bomb.

At this point, Officer Steve Matthews arrived—a sharp cop, a former member of our DSWAT Team, and now a member of the Repeat Offenders Unit, plainclothes officers who target repeat, violent offenders. Matthews looked around and was debating whether to get out his M4 rifle. He decided there were enough guns around and instead grabbed his high-speed surveillance camera. He took the first picture of Lee, who was visible through the lobby glass, and immediately forwarded this picture to arriving SWAT personnel, bomb techs, and the command bus.

The picture provided critical intel because it showed Lee's device and what appeared to be a lanyard around his neck. We had quickly identified the suspect because security at the Discovery building and MCPD officers from the 3rd District Station were familiar with him. On numerous occasions, Lee had protested outside the Discovery building, voicing concerns about overpopulation and the environment. He believed that through excessive reproduction and war, humans were destroying the Earth and that human

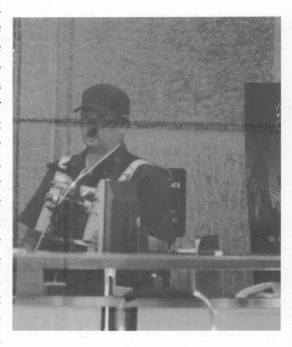

Suicide bomber James Lee with PBIED
(Courtesy of Steve Matthews, MCPD)

sterilization was the remedy. He asserted that the Discovery Channel's choice of programming promoted destructive human behavior.

Lee maintained the website SaveThePlanetProtest.com/protest.htm.

He was a disciple of Daniel Quinn, whose book *My Ishmael* suggests saving the planet the same way we created the Industrial Revolution—by people building on one another's inventive ideas. At core, Lee thought that people must live without giving birth to what he deemed "filthy human children" with new births that were polluting the planet. By reducing the human population, he could save the environment and the remaining species.

Lee had prior arrests for alien smuggling and disorderly conduct. Ironically, in 2008, the arresting officer at the Discovery building for disorderly conduct was Paden, who provided the initial description of Lee's device via the camera system.

When I arrived on scene as the SWAT commander, I joined Paden in the security office adjacent to a corridor at the back side of the lobby, behind a wall where Lee was located. It had a sophisticated camera system that the security officer manning the station could manipulate and adjust. The security officer Jackie Love remained at the cameras during the entire incident at great risk to herself. She did an outstanding job of adjusting the cameras to provide real-time intel and an opportunity to study Lee's device, the suspect, the hostages, and the layout of the lobby.

I immediately replaced the two IATs with two SWAT Assault Teams that we staged out of Lee's sight at the two corridors in the rear of the lobby—to prevent Lee from penetrating farther into the building. The back of the lobby where the two corridors were located was on the Delta side. I designated the Assault Team staged at the corridor closest to the Charlie/Delta corner as Delta One Assault Team and the corresponding passageway as the Delta One corridor (northwest corner). Clouser led this Assault Team.

The Assault Team staged near the security office with cameras at the Alpha/Delta corner was designated the Delta Two Assault Team and that relative corridor Delta Two (northeast corner). This team was led by Dillman. Each Assault Team had a sergeant and five officers.

I instructed Dillman and Clouser to develop a Deliberate Assault Plan and an Emergency Assault Plan with assistance from two experienced Central Team operators: Rob Kamensky and Steve Browne. Kamensky, a sniper, had brought both his .308-caliber sniper rifle and his .223-caliber M4. Kamensky would explore the interior sniper shot options, and if none were available, he could serve as an assaulter with his M4. Browne was well versed in close-quarters battle tactics. Having learned the value of delegating authority in a fast-moving dynamic situation, I was fortunate to have senior operators in whom I had great confidence.

While the assault plans were being developed, I brought a bomb tech from the Fire Marshal's Office into the security office to start gathering intel and assess the device. In addition, I brought in Ulisney, the former SEAL. I wanted his input, given his background in explosives, and even more importantly an assessment, given his overseas experience in the Navy. In December 1990, a violent war had broken out between armed militants and the Somali government. The capital, Mogadishu, was engulfed in violence. Ulisney had been part of a SEAL unit sent in January of 1991 during Operation Eastern Exit, the code name for evacuation of the U.S. embassy in Mogadishu. Our forces successfully evacuated 281 diplomats and civilians from 30 countries.

While we were developing assault plans and assessing Lee's device, I deployed three sniper teams. They use a system known as "clock and distance" to report their position to command—that is, the relative direction of an object using the analogy of a twelve-hour clock to describe angles and directions. Using this analogy, twelve o'clock means ahead or above, three o'clock means right, six o'clock means behind/below, and nine o'clock means to the left. The other eight hours refer to directions that are not directly in line with the four cardinal directions.

The distance is how far in yards or meters from the sniper's location to the target, usually determined through the use of a range finder. Once in position, the sniper team will communicate to Command its clock and distance to target. For example, "ten at sixty-five" means at the ten o'clock position and sixty-five yards to the target. Using this system, Command and all tactical operators know the location of each sniper team.

Table 2 illustrates the positioning of our law enforcement sniper teams, whose primary mission is to provide intelligence and, if circumstances require, eliminate the threat.

Within the first thirty minutes of SWAT being on scene, numerous tactical elements provided containment. Three sniper teams were deployed at clock and distance of 7/64, 9/46, and 11/56. The two Assault Teams, Delta One and Two, were concealed behind the back side of the lobby. The bomb techs integrated with SWAT and were gathering intel via the camera system. The tactical medics had also established a casualty collection point and were coordinating with fire and rescue. In addition, two BearCat tactical response armored personnel carriers (APCs), with tactical officers, were deployed outside the lobby to support the perimeter positions.

We staged other officers and DSWAT Sergeant Matt Domer and his K9 partner, a German Shepherd named Dallas, along the back hallway wall behind where Lee was located. Dallas had been specially trained and integrated with our SWAT Team to support our missions. Noise discipline was critical during this incident because we did not want to reveal our positions to the suspect. Dallas didn't make a sound the entire time, and his discipline proved invaluable.

The MSP SWAT Team, with which we had a great relationship, had just arrived. They have always been there when we needed them, including the three weeks in October 2002 during the hunt for the DC snipers, Malvo and Muhammad.

I asked their commander, Keith Runk, to establish a security corridor from the rear of our Assault Teams' position to a safe location farther within the building. If Lee released any hostages, we would funnel them back through the security corridor to the MSP SWAT Team. All released hostages would be treated as an "unknown" and handcuffed, searched, and then debriefed.

Table 2. Sniper Team Positioning During the

Discovery Hostage Incident

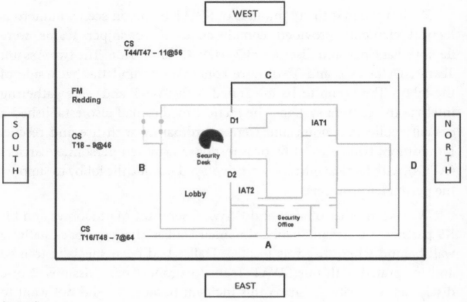

Legend

CS—Sniper Team's position at clock and distance: e.g., T16/48 are call signs for two SWAT Officers; 7@64 means they are at the 7 o'clock position and 64 yards from the target

Embedding—Captain Redding Bomb Tech position

Shortly thereafter, the FBI's Baltimore Field Office SWAT Team arrived. I knew their team leader, R. J. Porath. He inquired: "What do you need us to do?" I asked him and his team to clear the rest of the building and make sure there were no other threats. Our Code Red Teams had just started this task and were evacuating employees from the building. The FBI SWAT Team and our Code Red Teams began systematically clearing and evacuating the rest of the building in coordination with Discovery security. Ultimately, they would successfully evacuate 1,900 employees and fifty kids from a day care center.

Porath shared some critical information: The second hostage, McNulty, had had a rolling briefcase with him when he entered the lobby. That briefcase was now unattended on the lobby floor. I did not know this. What I did know was that Lee had brought a backpack into the lobby that was now unattended. This incident had all the appearances of a planned event in which a common practice is to bring secondary explosive devices. My fear was that Lee's backpack contained a timed IED. If so, that meant with every passing moment, we were nearing the time of detonation.

With McNulty, we now had a wild card. I had been watching him via the camera system, and he had all the appearances of being a true hostage. He was wearing tan pants and a polo-style, short-sleeve shirt. He did not appear to have anything under his clothing. However, we were not going to take any chances and had a special protocol for dealing with McNulty.

It was absolutely imperative that under no circumstance would we allow Lee to break containment. Every officer on scene, including a dozen or more bomb techs, believed Lee's explosive device was real. Under no circumstances could we allow Lee to break containment and wander the streets of downtown Silver Spring with an explosive device.

So that there would be no hesitation in SWAT officers on scene using deadly force, I announced over the police radio: "Under no circumstances will Lee be allowed to break containment. We will operate off our department's deadly force policy." MCPD Directive Function Code 131, Use of Force, says: "Officers may use deadly force to defend themselves or another person from what they have reasonable cause to perceive as an immediate threat of death or serious physical injury." This directive allows all MCPD officers to use deadly force to prevent loss of innocent lives during performance of their duties. I also wanted to make it clear that if an officer used deadly force under these circumstances, I would take responsibility for the order.

Once we contained Lee to the lobby, the preferred strategy was to negotiate release of the hostages and his surrender. If Lee attempted to exit the lobby doors or breached glass on the Alpha or Charlie side to break free, snipers had priority for use of deadly force, and if he attempted to escape via a corridor in the back of the lobby, the Assault Teams had the same priority.

Early on, bomb techs provided critical intel on the device. In their best estimation, it was real. Lee also appeared to have a positive block safety (attached to the lanyard)—identified from the first picture taken by Matthews. It also appeared that Lee was intensely gripping a firing device known as a dead-man switch. If he released or dropped the dead man grip, the explosive device would immediately detonate. Bomb techs believed that if the positive block were inserted into the device, it would prevent the dead-man switch from releasing and detonating.

Numerous bomb techs from the Montgomery County Fire and Rescue and the Fire Marshal's Office had been studying the device acutely from multiple locations. One bomb tech was with SWAT in the security office on the same level as the lobby behind a wall near the suspect as we watched him via the camera system. Captain Mike Redding, another bomb tech, was observing Lee through the lobby glass from a safe position with binoculars. He was near the Bravo/Charlie corner (southwest). Several other bomb techs were also observing from a second, larger security office via the camera system in the basement of another wing, a safe location far from the lobby.

As noted earlier, the bomb techs on site thought that the PBIED was real and that the suspect did have a dead-man switch. They believed that if Lee inserted the positive block safety, the device would not detonate. Their best estimate was that if the device detonated, it would cause significant damage to the lobby, including an incendiary effect and fragmentation that would kill or seriously injure everyone in the lobby area. They advised that the damage would be limited to the lobby area and would not travel up through the floors above and were confident there was no risk of a building collapse.

A concern I had was that the back wall of the south lobby was drywall, and we had many officers hidden on the other side of that wall. I asked if the device detonated, could potential fragmentation travel laterally, penetrate the drywall, and injure or kill officers? He said fragmentation going up was not an issue with concrete separating the different floors. The drywall, he said, was "dicey." I appreciated his honest response.

As a SWAT commander, I had to make decisions based on the best intel available at the time. We had probable cause to believe that the device was real. Probable cause is the standard, not 100% confirmation. There are only two ways to determine 100% if the device is real: 1) The suspect detonates it, or 2) after the incident, we send the device to the FBI Lab at Quantico, Virginia, for examination.

We had developed a number of tactical contingencies based on potential outcomes: surrender, a sniper option, Deliberate Assault, and Emergency Assault. First, our preference was surrender, for which we had a specific protocol. The suspect and three hostages were all near the security desk in the lobby. Lee was standing behind the desk, and security guard Fisher was to his right four feet slightly behind him. Wood and McNulty, the other two hostages, were still lying prone on the floor. The security desk favored the Charlie side (west) of the lobby.

For us to accept Lee's surrender, he would first have to release the hostages to the other side of the lobby. We would move the three hostages to the Alpha side (east) of the lobby away from Lee. We would bring two hostages—absent the wild card, McNulty—back through the corridor where the Delta Two Assault Team was staged. We treat all hostages as unknowns, so they would be instructed to put their hands on their heads and walk back to the corridor. There they would handcuffed and passed off to MSP SWAT, who would search them and take them to an isolated location within the building for debriefing by investigators.

There was a special protocol for wild-card McNulty. He would be instructed to remove his clothing. He would then be instructed to turn around 360 degrees so that we could visually confirm that he had no IEDs or weapons. We would then bring him back through the corridor and secure him as we did the two previous hostages.

For us to accept Lee's surrender, he first would have to insert the positive block safety into the dead-man switch and make the device safe. We would then order him through a set of additional safety protocols by requiring him to place the following items sequentially on the floor: the dead-man switch, his PBIED mounted on the Alice pack, what appeared to be a pipe bomb strapped to his right leg, and a handgun in his right rear pocket. He would then be told to remove any other devices or weapons he had on him and place them on the floor. Upon compliance, Lee would be told to move to the Alpha (east) side of the lobby, as the hostages had previously done. He would be instructed to remove all of his clothing and turn around 360 degrees. If all appeared clear, he would be directed back to the corridor and handcuffed and secured by MCPD SWAT. He would be turned over to uniformed officers and investigators for further action.

If the surrender option failed and we had to go to a tactical resolution, our preference would be a sniper shot. This option would give us precision fire and distance from the target, which is preferred when dealing with an explosive device. Ultimately, we eliminated the sniper option for a variety of reasons. We would only have used it if the suspect attempted to break containment by exiting the building out of the south lobby doors or if he broke through the lobby glass on the Alpha (east) or Charlie (west) side.

One reason we eliminated the sniper-shot option was that the glass at the Discovery building was thought to be hurricane glass, an impact-resistant glass designed to withstand pressure and strong hurricane winds. It is laminated glass and has two sheets of glass bonded with a protective interlayer. Hurricane glass can change the flight of a bullet once the round breaches the glass.

In a perfect world, during a sniper shot, we want the suspect to be within three to five feet of the glass. Depending on which sniper took the shot, once the round breached the glass, it would still have to travel an additional fifty-four to seventy-two feet within the lobby to reach Lee.

Ideally, we also wanted snipers to have a straight-on shot through the glass. The only sniper team with a straight-on shot from the nine o'clock position would have to shoot through two sets of glass on the double south lobby doors. Sniper teams covering the Alpha and Charlie sides had poor angles to glass to hit Lee. Their positioning was needed if Lee attempted to break glass and exit on the Alpha or Charlie side. Another concern was that there were numerous objects—artifacts and displays—suspended from the ceiling, all of which could cause a missed shot if the sniper did not observe them.

Kamensky, our senior sniper, explored the option of taking an interior sniper shot from the Delta One corridor. Our sniper rifles were .308-caliber Sakos equipped with 4.5X14 Leupold scopes and a mil dot reticle. The mil dot estimates range and target size and helps compensate for wind drift. The mil dots on a sniper rifle appear on both the vertical and horizontal crosshairs.

The interior shot would be only ten yards away, and even with the scope dialed down to its lowest power setting, the field of vision would be very limited. Lee's head would be all the sniper would see through the scope at a minimum setting. The concern was that the hostages would be facing the sniper as he took the shot. If the hostages reacted or moved laterally, the sniper would not be able to pick it up quickly and efficiently. We eliminated the interior sniper shot for these reasons. We felt that our .223-caliber M4 carbines would be effective at that range and would give the shooter a full field of vision.

Kamensky even explored the option of taking a sniper shot through the ceiling rafters, but he determined that option was not feasible. In 2011, Kamensky won the invitational sniper team competition at Fort Meade with Officer Wayne Hoyt, so I always trusted his judgment. Though the sniper resolution was our preferred tactical option absent surrender, it was not viable.

Our next preferred option if it went to a tactical resolution was a Deliberate Assault executed by our two Assault Teams staged out of sight behind a wall at the rear of the lobby. A Deliberate Assault is a proactive movement executed at the moment of greatest tactical opportunity. To initiate a Deliberate Assault, we wanted to observe four factors: 1) the positive block safety be engaged in the dead-man switch and the device made safe; 2) favorable positioning of the hostages; 3) Lee be at the desk with his back to the Assault Teams, particularly the Delta One Assault Team because it would initiate the assault; and 4) ideally but not absolutely necessary, that Lee be distracted and engaged in conversation on the phone.

The Assault Teams were also prepared to do an Emergency Assault executed by SWAT to prevent the immediate loss of life. Factors may not favor a successful outcome at the moment SWAT executes an emergency action. This is our least-preferred tactical option because historically it has a very low probability of success. Unlike the proactive Deliberate Assault, the Emergency Assault is often a reactive response.

I now met with the two Assault Team Leaders, Dillman and Clouser, and Officers Browne and Kamensky to discuss the Deliberate and Emergency Assault Plans that they had developed.

Under the Deliberate Assault Plan, by watching the suspect via the camera system, I could determine if the four factors we wanted existed. Under the deliberate option, the Delta One Assault Team would initiate action. Using the security cam, I could advise the shooters that the suspect's back was to them and give updates as they covertly moved into position. With the suspect's back to Delta One, three shooters would move stealth to the threshold of the lobby at the Delta One corridor. Under no circumstance would they penetrate into the lobby.

The Delta One corridor was wide enough to accommodate three shooters online (side by side). Ideally, we wanted to get three shooters online so they could execute simultaneous fire—the same tactic that Navy SEALs used during the rescue of Captain Richard Phillips in April 2009 when Somali pirates hijacked the cargo ship *MV Maersk Alabama* and took him hostage. The SEALs' task was far more complicated because they had to take out three different subjects simultaneously with three shooters who were shooting from a moving boat at a moving boat and through glass. In contrast, we had to take out one subject with three shooters. If we were compromised while moving into position, any shooter had the authority to take the shot.

Clouser was rotating three shooters in this position, all experienced SWAT officers: Kamensky, John McGaha, and Kendrick Stephens. Each man would stay on gun in the Number 1 position for fifteen minutes and then rotate back to the rear to keep the team fresh. Kamensky noted that from a certain angle, you could see Lee's reflection off the lobby glass while remaining undetected.

A great concern was that when Lee went down, he would be out of view of the Delta One Assault Team if he went down inside or on the other side of the desk. They would not be in position to deliver follow-up shots if needed.

The Delta Two Assault Team would move immediately upon hearing Delta One's first shot. We could script the entry of Delta Two because we would know Lee's location via the camera system. The first two Delta Two Team members would do a limited penetration into the lobby to their right until they had a view of Lee. They would deliver follow-up shots if needed. The third and fourth members would go left, covering their backs if we had missed anything on the camera.

The Emergency Assault Plan was similar. Delta One assignments were the same: Under no circumstances would Delta One ever enter or break the lobby threshold. Delta Two would always be the flanking team. The positioning of the two Assault Teams formed a tactical "L" so that the entire lobby area would be covered by overlapping and interlocking fields of fire.

Under both options, all shots were to be to the head only. We did not want to risk hitting the device and detonating it. There was a "no survival clause," meaning that if it went to a tactical resolution, we would continue shooting Lee until all movement ceased. We could not risk the suspect detonating the device because casualties to the hostages and SWAT would be catastrophic.

Under no circumstances for any of the assault contingencies were any SWAT personnel to approach the suspect after he was eliminated. SWAT would withdraw and turn the scene over to the bomb techs for Render Safe Procedures (RSPs).

About two hours into the incident, all the stars lined up. The bomb techs advised that it appeared Lee had inserted the positive block safety into the dead-man switch, rendering the device safe. Lee had inserted it on previous occasions, but it had only remained in a few seconds, and then he quickly removed it. This time, it remained. Lee was talking on the phone to negotiators and, I think, forgot that the positive block safety was still in the device. In addition to the positive block safety being in the firing device, the hostages were in favorable positions, so we had clear shooting lanes. Lee was standing at the security desk, half facing

McNulty, who was now standing on the other side of the desk and half facing the security guard, Fisher, who was several feet to Lee's right behind the security desk. Wood was still lying prone on the floor in view of Lee.

Lee's back was to Delta One. He was on the speaker phone with negotiators, threatening to harm the hostages. We could hear the conversation from the other side of the wall, and I was watching via the camera system.

With the four factors that we wanted now in play, I brought Delta Two Team Leader Dillman and members of his team into the security office so they could observe the positioning of Lee and the hostages. I then walked down the back hallway to the Delta One Team Leader, Clouser. Clouser had drawn a diagram of the lobby and security desk on the wall with a magic marker. He then drew the position of Lee and the hostages as I detailed their locations. He then began to bring members of his team to view the layout and current positioning of suspect and hostages.

While this was occurring, I got on the police radio with Command. I advised them that all the factors we were looking for to do a Deliberate Assault were in play and requested permission to execute the action. After a brief pause, Command responded: "You have authority for the Deliberate Assault." I acknowledged Command and advised all SWAT units to "stand by for a Deliberate Assault." I would give the order from the security office because, using the cameras, I could confirm that nothing had changed and make sure that Lee's back was to Delta One as I gave the order. It took me about ten seconds to walk quietly and briskly back to the security office. I viewed the cameras, and the bomb techs confirmed that the positive block safety was still in the device. It appeared nothing had changed. I was reaching for the microphone to give the order over the radio to initiate the assault when Command came on the air and said, "Stand by on the Deliberate Assault." I immediately responded to Command, "I can't emphasize enough what it means if we lose this moment of opportunity."

Command responded: "Stand by."

Again, I reiterated, "I can't emphasize enough what it means if we lose this moment of opportunity." Again, "stand by." Command wanted to ensure the floors above the lobby had been evacuated. I acknowledged in frustration.

Command officials later explained they were worried about what would happen if bomb techs were wrong in their estimation of damage should the device detonate. They wanted to play it safe.

About five minutes later, Lee ordered all of the hostages to move close to him around the desk. Bomb techs advised that it appeared that he had removed the positive block safety from the dead-man switch. I thought that this was it. I was greatly concerned that he was going to release the dead-man switch and detonate his device. Fortunately, he did not.

Lee would not reinsert the positive block safety into the dead-man switch for the remainder of the event. From that moment forward, SWAT lost the initiative. We had become reactive instead of proactive. After ten minutes, Command advised, "If the suspect reinserts the positive block safety, you have authority for the Deliberate Assault."

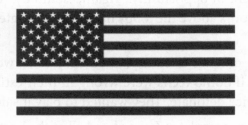

7. Discovery Hostage Rescue

Duty Calls

S oon thereafter, Command received information that Lee had multiple bombs on his person and in a bag. He had been planning this event for three to four years.

Negotiations continued. John Wilkes, MCPD's most senior negotiator, was the primary negotiator talking to Lee on the speaker phone. The circumstances that led to Wilkes becoming the primary negotiator with Lee were comical. Wilkes was a firearms instructor and was at the outdoor range in Poolesville when the ERT callout alerted him on his pager. Poolesville and Silver Spring are at opposite ends of Montgomery County, twenty-eight miles apart, so Wilkes knew he would be the last of the negotiating team to arrive. He explained that typically, early on, they designate one of the first arriving negotiators as primary negotiator, and he is supported by a coach. Negotiators arriving later are usually given tasks of gathering intel to support the negotiations.

While en route, he received a phone call from the head of the negotiating team, Lieutenant Ron Smith, who asked that Wilkes call a particular phone number hoping a Discovery supervisor would answer a list of questions for Wilkes to ask. He is a very humble guy and a total team player, so he said, "Sure, LT, whatever you need."

Wilkes called the number, and someone answered. Wilkes identified himself by saying, "This is John Wilkes with the MCPD." The person on the other end of the line started yelling, ranting, and raving. Wilkes was stunned. He realized immediately that he was talking to Lee. Apparently, the number John called also rang at the security desk, and Lee answered the phone and put it on speaker. Wilkes quickly regained his composure and began talking to Lee.

This was how Wilkes, who had no expectation of being the primary negotiator, fell into that role. The negotiators were hopeful that they could achieve a peaceful resolution. Factors that they viewed as favorable were that Discovery was not a government, religious, or symbolic building. The hostage taker was in a prominent, visible location in the lobby, and a significant period of time had elapsed with no injury to the hostages. They viewed Lee as an activist, and when Lee had been arrested there in the past, he had not resisted.

As negotiations began between Lee and Wilkes, SWAT could hear the interaction from the lobby speaker phone because we were covertly staged on the other side of the lobby's back wall. Wilkes tried to get Lee to empathize with the hostages. He also attempted to humanize the hostages. Wilkes was very patient, but despite his best efforts, it became clear that Lee was suicidal. He was negative toward the hostages and himself. Negotiations had been ongoing for a long time. Here is an excerpt from those negotiations as the incident neared its conclusion:

Wilkes: "Mr. Lee, as I said earlier, I am not bullshitting. I am trying to be as honest as I can."

Lee interrupted and yelled: "Police lie; I know the police lie. I dealt with you all the time. You are patronizing me; tell me who do you think you are!"

Wilkes: "Mr. Lee, I am not patronizing you. I swear I am not patronizing you."

Lee: "Yes, you are. Then why are you not in touch with the Discovery Channel?"

Wilkes: "We are trying, as we speak, to get in touch with Discovery Channel executives."

Lee: "Well, great. If you are talking to me, how come you are not talking to them?"

Wilkes: "We have other officers who are in contact with or trying to contact Discovery executives so you can air your grievances. We are doing this on multiple fronts. I have decided to call you because we want to help you resolve this peacefully and work with you to help you get some of your issues resolved. Let's do this; let's release those people in the lobby."

Lee angrily interrupted: "Oh, stop bullshitting me, man. As soon as I release them, you will take a sniper to my head! When you have gotten my demands met, we will talk about releasing people. All right!"

Wilkes: "What about the people in the lobby? Look what you are putting them through."

Lee: "They mean nothing to me. All right."

Wilkes: "They have families. They have loved ones."

Lee: "I don't give a shit! What I care about is the company [Discovery] stop broadcasting these shows that will make people have families. Don't you listen to me? Don't you listen to me?"

Wilkes: "Mr. Lee, I have been listening to everything you have said."

Lee: "Well, then, just stop having families. This guy [hostage] has two kids over here, for crying out loud. Who told him to have kids?"

Wilkes: "I've become concerned about you, but I am also concerned about these poor people in the lobby. I mean—"

Lee interrupted yet again: "No one is innocent! Everyone is filth, all right! We need to stop people breeding more filth. I don't care about their families. I care about what I asked for. So don't tell me that shit. I have no sympathy."

Wilkes: "It sounds to me that you are pretty passionate about your beliefs, and it sounds to me you don't want to hurt anyone today. Is that what I'm hearing?"

Lee: "People will get hurt, all right, and the whole world will see it."

Wilkes: "Then you're not going to get your grievances dealt with."

Lee: "I don't care. I'll be dead, all right!"

Wilkes: "Look, I don't want you dead, Mr. Lee. I want—"

Lee interrupted: "If I blow up, I won't care!"

Wilkes: "Mr. Lee, how are you going to get your grievances dealt with if you're dead? That is going to accomplish nothing."

Lee: "Everyone will know I was talking serious when I said that."

Wilkes: "Hey, Mr. Lee—"

Lee interrupted: "What the hell is wrong with you, man?"

Wilkes: "Mr. Lee, if you look out the lobby, I think everybody is taking you serious. I mean everybody."

Lee: "I don't see anybody taking me serious."

Wilkes: "I mean everybody is here because we take you serious. If we didn't think you were serious, we wouldn't be out here in the numbers we are today."

Lee: "I see a few dozen."

Wilkes: "No, Mr. Lee, there are hundreds of us here, hundreds. The media is here; I mean everybody is here. You've got a wide audience. I wouldn't be surprised if this was being broadcasted across the country. You have an audience; this is your opportunity with this audience in front of you to deal with this. Okay? I mean, where else are you going to find an audience like this? Mr. Lee, you haven't hurt anyone."

Lee: "Not yet. I am not going to do a half-ass job. Either I get my way, or I am going to die today. All right!"

Wilkes: "You have to admit it's tough for us when you have a bomb strapped to you. You have innocent people in the lobby and you—"

Lee interrupted: "I don't see any innocent people. You understand: No one is innocent; no one is innocent."

Wilkes: "Mr. Lee, I am not going to bullshit you. We are not here to use violence against you; we have not—"

Lee interrupted: "You're going to kill me. I know what you are going to do."

Wilkes: "Mr. Lee, we are not going to kill you."

Meanwhile, Dillman, the Delta Two Assault Team leader, was rotating members of the Assault Team through the various positions for bathroom breaks and to keep the team fresh. Mercurio, a member of the Assault Team, recalled his thoughts at that time. It was clear to him that Lee did not want a peaceful resolution. To Mercurio, Lee seemed to get angrier and angrier by the moment. On multiple occasions, Mercurio and teammate Ed Clarke whispered to each other that the hostages were in grave danger and that SWAT would have to resolve the situation. Mercurio was wondering what was in the tanks and concerned about the dead-man switch and the consequences if it was released. He asked God several times to make sure his aim was true and that his children would not lose their father on this day.

The members of the assault teams wore black combat fatigues, black shirts, lightweight boots, and ballistic helmets and had on heavy body armor with a large emblem with the word POLICE on the front and back that was clearly visible. They were also equipped with Peltor ComTac tactical headsets, which are designed for military and SWAT operations and provide communication and ear protection from noise as well. Tactical operators were armed with M4 carbines and .45-caliber semi-automatic pistols as their backup weapons.

Dillman shared his professional and personal thoughts while waiting to execute the tactical assault. He said it was very clear to him early on that this incident was going to be resolved by SWAT, not negotiation. We had plenty of personnel, and he could have easily had another SWAT officer replace him as part of the assault team. Knowing the risk factor, in good conscience, he could not ask men to go into harm's way without being part of that team. While waiting, he received a couple of phone calls from his twelve-year-old son Cole, who saw the events unfolding on TV. Cole was concerned that his father would be too busy to take him to football practice, where Dillman served as a coach for the team.

Dillman played down the magnitude of the event and said it was unlikely he would make it home in time to take him to practice. He wondered if this would be the last conversation his son would ever have with his father. Dillman had become increasingly frustrated with Command because it seemed apparent, as more time passed, that the incident was going to be resolved by an Emergency Assault. He didn't want the lives of Assault Team members left to chance and was concerned about the impact on their families if serious injury or loss of life occurred.

Three hours and fifty-five minutes into the incident, one of our snipers, Spiro Tatakis, reported that it appeared the security guard, Fisher, was giving hand signals to the other two hostages. I thought I had observed this on the camera system as well, but I wasn't sure. I asked: "Are you absolutely sure?" Tatakis responded: "No doubt."

It seemed that the hostages were going to take some sort of action, though what that action would be we did not know. Based on these observations, I came on the air, advised Command of the situation, and told our Assault Teams to be prepared for an Emergency Assault.

Moments later, I suddenly heard a lot of commotion on the other side of the wall. Lee ran from behind the security desk and momentarily disappeared from camera view. There was no doubt in my mind that it was going down, and I immediately came on the police radio and ordered: "Emergency Assault, Emergency Assault. GO, GO, GO!"

To the credit of the two Assault Team leaders, Dillman and Clouser, each had immediately reacted when they had heard the disturbance and initiated an Emergency Assault. There was no delay between the order being given and the movement of the Assault Teams. All was simultaneous, reaffirming we were all on the same page as to what action we needed to take.

What was actually occurring was the three hostages were all making a break and attempting to run for safety, and Lee was in pursuit.

The Delta One Assault Team was moving through the Delta One corridor and would not break the threshold of the lobby. The first SWAT officer was McGaha, who observed Lee running laterally, from left to right, on the opposite side of the security desk pursuing two hostages.

McGaha was about to take the shot with his M4 carbine when the security guard, Fisher, ran directly at McGaha into his line of fire. He "checked" his fire, grabbed the security officer, and passed him off to other officers down the line. Other officers secured Fisher and threw him into a closet.

The Number 2 person was Stephens. He quickly acquired Lee in his EOTech sight and fired at the suspect with his Colt Commando M4 carbine. We later determined that one round struck the top of the metal Alice pack frame that Lee was wearing; it contained the PBIED. The round did not penetrate the steel bar at the base of Lee's neck and grazed off, causing a flesh wound to his neck. The impact prompted Lee to reach up with his right hand to the back of his neck. This caused his body to turn slightly to his right. Stephens later commented that he thought that first shot would be his last act on this Earth.

Stephens, McGaha, and other members of Delta One were careful not to penetrate into the threshold of the lobby as has been detailed in the assault plans.

Simultaneously, the Delta Two Assault Team moved into position. Mercurio and Dave Reed entered through the Delta Two corridor along with other members of their team. They proceeded to their right and came "online" as stipulated in the Emergency Assault Plan. Mercurio, the Number 1 person into the lobby, observed Lee pursuing two hostages. Mercurio immediately opened fire. He recalled the suspect looking over at him with an agitated expression on his face, and then Mercurio pulled the trigger. He said he never heard the shot. The round hit Lee, and the suspect started to drop to the floor when the Number 2 person, Reed, struck Lee with multiple rounds. Mercurio dropped to a knee to deliver additional rounds, being careful not to hit the tanks. Both officers struck Lee with multiple rounds. The second hostage, Wood, ran out the lobby doors and was secured unharmed by perimeter officers. The third hostage, McNulty, ran behind a concrete pillar in the lobby and took cover. Suddenly, amid all the gunfire, he made a mad dash for the lobby doors, causing Mercurio and Reed to check their fire briefly so as to not hit the hostage who had now appeared in their backdrop. The hostage made it safely out the lobby doors and was secured by perimeter officers. Once the hostage was safely out of their backdrop, Reed and

Mercurio quickly fired additional rounds, fearing Lee could still activate the device.

Two other SWAT officers, Clarke and Jordan Young, had entered through the Delta Two corridor and cleared the area to the left, covering the backs of Reed and Mercurio. Clarke recalls that by the time we cleared the area behind them, the incident was pretty much resolved. The Element Leader, Browne, while not actively engaged, came online with Reed and Mercurio, directing the shooters not to over-penetrate.

After giving the Emergency Assault order, I ran down the back hallway and fell in behind the Delta One Assault Team at the Delta One corridor to coordinate activity. Lee was down and had been hit sixteen times at this point from .223-caliber rounds fired from M4s. I knew that Dillman was with Delta Two, so I thought it prudent to join Delta One. I advised Command that Lee was down.

Clouser detected movement from Lee and advised: "He is still moving. Does anyone have a shot?" No response from any tactical officers. One of Lee's hands could be seen twitching. The concern was that as long as Lee was alive, he could detonate the device, which would be catastrophic for all of us in the lobby area. Delta One was not in a position to deliver a follow-up shot because the security desk blocked its view.

Lee had gone down in the forward part of the lobby near the lobby doors. His feet were now facing toward the rear of the lobby with his head in the direction of the south lobby doors. The Alice pack had slid up high on his body, partially obscuring his head from the Assault Teams' view.

We had preached headshots only, and it became apparent that nobody had the shot.

The Delta Two leader, Dillman, called out, "Moving," in an effort to position himself for a headshot. "Moving" is a request to move from one position to another. It must be acknowledged by another tactical officer in proximity before any movement may occur.

Clouser, realizing that Dillman was positioning himself for a final follow-up shot, acknowledged, "Move." Dillman proceeded to the front lobby area along the Alpha side to deliver a headshot.

While this was occurring, an officer still online from the Delta Two flanking team, taking cover behind a concrete pillar, fired one round in an attempt to deliver the final shot. The round struck one of the yellow PBIED tanks. There was a pop and a hiss and release of a gaseous substance. Fortunately, there was no detonation. We all breathed a sigh of relief. We would learn later that the yellow tanks contained MAPP gas, which requires a significant heat source to ignite. The round fired from the outside did not create enough heat to ignite the MAPP gas and cause the device to detonate.

Dillman reached his position, called, "Shot," to alert the team and fired one round to Lee's head, at which point all movement from Lee ceased. I then advised Command that the suspect had been eliminated, that all three hostages had been rescued unharmed, and that no SWAT officer had sustained injuries. I advised SWAT teams to withdraw and indicated that we would turn the scene over to the bomb techs for RSP.

Suddenly, unbelievably, Clouser advised that the suspect was still moving. One of Lee's hands was still twitching after he had been shot seventeen times. Maybe he was dead, and this was some sort of involuntary muscle response? I didn't know. We couldn't chance turning the scene over to the bomb techs until all movement ceased.

I ordered the Delta Two Assault Team to withdraw along with most members of Delta One. I followed the tactical principle of having a minimum number of people down range with an explosive device. In the worst-case scenario if things went bad, this practice would minimize police casualties. A single officer, Stephens, went into the lobby from the Delta One corridor and from behind a concrete pillar fired the final shot to Lee's head. All movement ceased—again! We waited ten minutes with no more movement from Lee. Stephens had the distinction of firing the first and last shots.

Tatakis was in a sniper position covering the Alpha side at the seven o'clock position sixty-five yards from Lee. He was across the street in a concealed position on the opposite side of Georgia Avenue, hidden behind a stack of outdoor furniture on an uninhabited restaurant patio. It was a hot day, ninety-five degrees, and he recalls a waitress opening the sliding glass door behind him slightly and whispering, "Hey, would you like a drink?" In a discreet fashion, so as to not compromise his position, she delivered drinks to both him and his observer. He thought how bizarre this was, sipping Pellegrino water, watching some "nut job" with hostages through his rifle scope. He recalls watching the Emergency Assault from his position through his scoped rifle. He observed the hostages make a run for it with Lee in pursuit. In an instant, he saw the SWAT Assault Teams enter the lobby. He saw the puffs of smoke from the SWAT officers' guns as they engaged the suspect and saw Lee fall to the ground out of his view. He said at that point he turned to his observer, Mike Powers, and said: "It's over, man; they got him. Let's get out of here." He packed up his gear and waited for the order to secure.

We were now satisfied that we could safely turn the scene over to the bomb techs.

Investigators and ballistic reports would later determine that four different SWAT officers had fired twenty rounds: Eighteen hit Lee, one round hit a yellow tank, and one was a miss. Five shots hit Lee in the head, eleven rounds struck his torso on the right side of his body between the gap in the canisters of the explosive device on Lee's person. Two rounds struck his right arm.

When Stephens fired the round that struck the Alice pack frame at the base of Lee's neck, it caused Lee to grab his neck with his right hand and spin slightly to his right. Lee's hand obscured his head. Mercurio, who was entering from the opposite corridor, later told me: "Sarge, I know you said headshots, but his hand obscured his head, so I transitioned from head to body shots." When Mercurio and Reed entered from the other corridor, they explained later, they fired multiple rounds to the torso that was exposed between the tanks of the PBIED. They did a great job of adjusting on the fly and taking the available shots. I was satisfied with our hit ratio because our assaulters were shooting on the move at a moving target. The shooters all did a good job of checking their fire when needed not to hit the hostages. The only questionable shot was the one that hit the yellow propane tank.

After securing the lobby area for the bomb tech RSP, I gathered the team in a hallway at a safe location. The team had executed an Emergency Assault that statistically had a very low probability of success. They had rescued the three hostages unharmed, eliminated the suspect, and incurred no police casualties. I told all assembled how proud I was of each of them.

I instructed our four shooters to keep their weapons as they were, with the selector switch in the "safe" position, for the investigators. I separated them from the team into their own room. I instructed the rest of the team to "gear down" in a conference room we had secured.

I then advised Runk, the MSP SWAT Team leader, that his team could secure from the site and thanked him for his prompt response.

I then met with Porath, leader of the FBI Baltimore Field Office SWAT Team, and thanked him for his team's response.

Our Code Red Teams, working with FBI SWAT and Discovery security personnel, safely evacuated over 1,900 civilians on that day and fifty kids from a day care facility.

Soon thereafter, investigators arrived, and after a debrief, they cleared us to go home. While driving home, Mercurio reflected on the day's events and called his wife to let her know he was all right. His daughter asked when he was coming home for dinner. He said she asked with all the innocence of a four-year-old and with no knowledge of what her dad had just experienced. It crushed him. He prayed to God and gave thanks to God and his team. Mercurio, a man of conscience, did an outstanding job on this day. The public often overlooks the fact that police officers have families and are people with feelings as well.

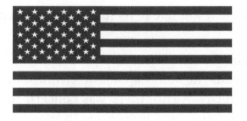

8. Discovery Aftermath

Fate

While our job in SWAT was over, the job of the bomb techs was just beginning. The SWAT operation had taken four hours; the bomb techs' job would take another twelve hours. All told, it was a sixteen-hour day for them.

The concern for the bomb techs was that the positive block safety was not in the firing device, and the PBIED should have detonated. There was a thought that maybe Lee's body position when he went down was in some way preventing the device from detonating.

Numerous bomb squads from the DC region had responded to assist the MCPD bomb techs, including Prince George's County, U.S. Capital, Metro Transit, FBI, and Virginia State Police.

The Virginia State Police bomb squad deployed with electronic countermeasures (ECM) equipment. It is one of the few bomb squads in the country designated with this capability. The ECM will shut down all radio traffic. It can be used to prevent the electronic detonation of an explosive device. Its use will also shut down all radio air traffic control with the FAA. There are numerous federal protocols to get its use approved; one bomb tech commented that its approval takes an act of God. Though officials approved ECM use, ultimately, we did not use it because the incident was late in its resolution and quickly moving to a tactical phase.

Captain Kevin Frazier was the commander of the Montgomery County Bomb Squad. The bomb squads determined that removal of Lee's device was the priority. Again, there was concern that his positioning may have created a "hang pin," preventing the device from going off.

Frazier coordinated bomb tech operations among the various agencies. Robot operations would complete the removal remotely. After removal, PAN disrupters would render the device safe in the lobby. A PAN disrupter is a non-electronic explosive ordinance tool to disable and render safe IEDs remotely without initiating them.

The final phase would then be the search of the suspect and the lobby.

Multiple robotic platforms were used in a joint coordinated effort by various agencies to cut away and remove devices from Lee's body. It was a lengthy, carefully orchestrated operation using two-man bomb tech teams from multiple jurisdictions rotated through RSPs.

Frazier indicated that they learned that bomb squads could simultaneously operate three robots wirelessly. However, when they introduced a fourth platform, everything shut down. They quickly resolved the issue by operating the fourth robot off a tether. The wireless robots entered through one lobby door and tethered a second.

The bomb techs also learned that some platforms were suited for particular tasks. The larger platforms performed well at flipping the body while smaller platforms were better suited to cut off the straps. Another issue was decontamination of the robots from Lee's bodily fluids in the aftermath.

While in the past the bomb squads usually trained on independent tasks, they quickly learned how to perform as a team working to perform a single task.

The primary device on the Alice frame contained four improvised incendiary devices (IIDs) and were all rendered safe. Bomb techs also rendered a fifth device, an IED pipe bomb, safe as well.

Once bomb techs cleared the lobby with robots and rendered the devices safe, they had to don their heavy bomb suits and physically clear the lobby. Simultaneous to the bomb tech operation in the lobby, twenty bomb-detection K9 dogs from multiple agencies swept the perimeter and other building areas searching for secondary devices; they found none. The entire bomb tech operation to clear and declare the building safe lasted about twelve hours.

Initially, investigators could not locate a residence for Lee. He had no registered vehicles, and two previous addresses were no longer valid. The morning after the incident, a desk clerk at an MCPD district station received a phone call from a person reporting that Lee had rented a room in his house. He asked the police to remove Lee's items because he wanted to make his house safe.

Investigators and bomb techs obtained and executed a search warrant for the residence. They found more devices and rendered them safe. They also found implements used to make the devices, detailed assembly instructions, bomb-making videos, and live pipe bombs.

Investigators also recovered a thumb drive with a narrated video showing Lee testing his explosive device in an isolated wooded area. The device detonated and was clearly functional.

The FBI Explosives Laboratory Division in Quantico did an assessment of Lee's IIDs and IED. What was each device, and was it functional? Here is the Reader's Digest version of the FBI report. The device was four IIDs (four yellow propane tanks filled with MAPP gas) designed to create an incendiary effect. Lee placed a red oxygen tank mounted in the middle of the yellow propane tanks to enhance the thermal effect of the MAPP gas. MAPP gas can reach 5,300 degrees Fahrenheit when mixed with oxygen. A pipe bomb attached to Lee's leg was the equivalent of a military fragmentation grenade that can cause death or serious injury to those within a twelve-meter radius. He wired all items in sequence so they would essentially detonate simultaneously.

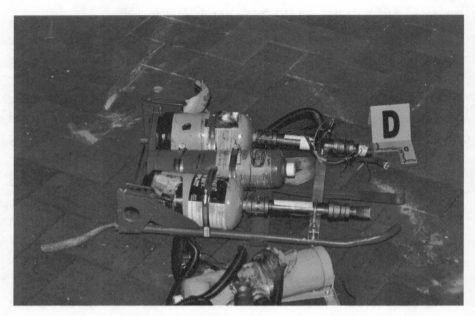

Person-borne improvised explosive device that James Lee was wearing during the Discovery incident

(Courtesy of MCPD)

The FBI Lab determined that the device was functional and that if the device had detonated, the resulting fire and explosion from the IIDs and IED would have caused death, personal injury, and property damage that was consistent with the estimate that the on-scene bomb techs had provided.

This determination raised a follow-up question: If the PBIED was functional and Lee had not inserted the positive block safety, why did the device fail to detonate?

Lee was a proficient and practiced bomb maker, but he had to go through a series of checks to arm his device. When he first entered the lobby, he fired several shots and took the security guard, Fisher, hostage. He then donned his device and began arming it. While going through the arming procedure, a second person, whom he took as a hostage, interrupted him, and he ordered the second hostage to lie prone on the ground. Lee returned to arming his device when a third person entered the lobby and broke his sequence once again. He also ordered this third hostage into a prone position on the floor. The interruptions caused Lee to forget to complete the final process of arming the device. He did not turn the dead-man switch power packs on, which would have armed the device. Despite his bomb-making skills, he was not a proficient and practiced hostage taker when under stress, which is why the device did not detonate that day.

One other reason occurs to me: God was on our side that day. Just like Samuel Jackson said in the movie Pulp Fiction after a scared kid fired multiple rounds at him and his partner, John Travolta, at point-blank range but did not hit either of them: "This was divine intervention." On August 9, 2010, Lee had posted in his Outlook calendar for September 1, 2010, the statement "The Final Day." He had come to Discovery to die. FBI investigators determined that Lee was a "lone wolf" domestic terrorist—the first suicide bomber with hostages in the U.S.

We learned many lessons that fateful day.

Best-Job Observation: Of all our law enforcement units responding that day, uniform patrol did the best job. Patrol quickly shut down and isolated an entire city block in a congested business district, diverting pedestrian and vehicle traffic and securing the perimeter. Under direction from Paden, two IATs were formed at Delta One and Two corridors. This prevented Lee from penetrating farther into the building. Paden also secured a high-value target: the security camera that provided real-time observation of Lee, the hostages, and the PBIED.

SWAT Lessons: We determined that our Code Red Teams' training when we integrated our bomb techs with the Code Red Teams before this incident was invaluable. As noted earlier, two months before the Discovery incident, we trained for an identical scenario: a suicide bomber with hostages. Both buildings were of similar size and design. Just by chance, when we did the suicide bomber scenario, it was in the building's lobby; as fate would have it, the actual incident was in the Discovery building's lobby.

In many traditional hostage situations, there is a concept that time can be an ally to police. There were some on the Command bus who felt that time was on our side. I did not agree. This incident had all the appearances of a planned event. Common practice in planned events involves secondary explosive devices. Lee had brought a bag into the lobby and left it unattended on the floor. My concern was that this bag could contain a secondary, timed explosive device, which would have meant that with every passing second, we were getting closer to the moment of detonation. The wild-card hostage, McNulty, introduced a second potential timed device with his rolling briefcase. From my perspective, the circumstances were quite different from a typical hostage situation.

New Mexico Tech subject-matter experts authorized release of the PBIED suicide bomber incident response protocol chart. Developed by individuals with comprehensive knowledge in the field, it recommends a course of action based on the particular circumstances in a PBIED suicide bomber incident. I was very familiar with the suggested protocols because I had studied them at length when developing our Code Red Teams (see Table 3).

Table 3. PBIED Suicide Bomber

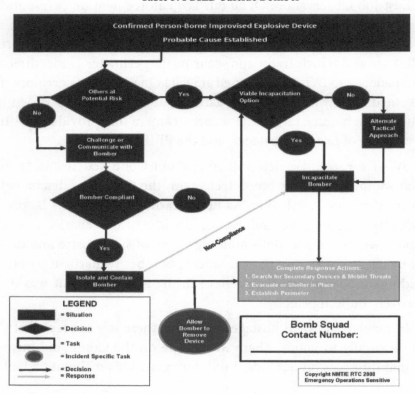

The first issue is to determine whether we believe there is a PBIED suicide bomber based on the totality of the circumstances. Every bomb tech and all law enforcement present on scene at Discovery believed the device to be real, so certainly probable cause existed that there was a PBIED suicide bomber. It is important to recognize that probable cause based on the "totality of the circumstances" is the standard, not 100% confirmation of an explosive device. The only way to have 100% confirmation is if the suspect detonates the explosive device or in the aftermath of an incident when it is sent to the FBI Laboratory in Quantico for analysis. Law enforcement can only act on its best information available at that time.

Negotiations and surrender are the preferred resolutions. We had a tactical contingency in place for surrender. However, protocol recommends that if others are at risk (certainly the hostages were) and a viable tactical option exists, we should use the tactical option to incapacitate the subject. When the bomb techs advised that Lee had inserted the positive block safety into the dead-man switch about two hours into the incident and the positive block safety remained in the device for an extended period of time, SWAT had a viable tactical option. At that moment, I believe Command should have allowed us to execute our Deliberate Assault Plan at the greatest moment of tactical advantage, when the positive block safety was in the firing device.

I received two explanations of why Command told us to stand down. One, noted above, was that Command wanted to confirm that floors above the lobby had been evacuated in case the bomb tech assessment of the device's destructive power was incorrect. The second was that some Command personnel thought we could still negotiate a resolution. My contention: When others are at risk and a viable tactical option exists and we choose to negotiate rather than execute a tactical option, we elevate the value of the suspect's life above those of the hostages.

Ultimately, the hostages took the initiative. The moment SWAT was ordered to stand down, SWAT became reactive, not proactive. Under our proactive Deliberate Assault Plan, SWAT would pick the moment of the assault, know the positioning of the suspect and hostages, and have many other factors in our favor. In contrast, the Emergency Assault

Plan was reactive, and instead of having static targets in known fixed positions, SWAT had running targets that it had to identify quickly. SWAT officers from each Assault Team had to check their fire to avoid hitting hostages on the run. During the Emergency Assault, SWAT lost positive control of the hostages, including the wild card, McNulty.

The Discovery building incident led to some equipment changes within SWAT. We were greatly concerned about how effective our .223-caliber ammunition was since Lee was still moving after seventeen hits on his body. Kamensky asked the FBI ballistic experts for input. Our Colt Commando M4 had 10.5-inch barrels and a barrel twist rate of 1:7. "Twist rate" refers to the rate of spin in the rifle barrel in inches per turn. It is important that the barrel has an adequate twist rate to stabilize the bullet as shooters fire. The round we used was federal 55 grain tactical bonded. The FBI ballistic experts suggested a slightly heavier round of 62 grains, a change we implemented immediately because guns with shorter barrels need added bullet mass to compensate for lost velocity.

We also didn't like the fact that we were not confident in taking an interior sniper shot at thirty feet because of the magnification settings of our Leupold scope. Kamensky identified an effective solution: LWRCI Rapid Engagement Precision Rifles (REPRs)—basically a .308-caliber M4. Each has a 1-4 power Nightforce scope with illuminated reticle. The REPR gives us a more effective round at close range, and the 1-4 power scope allows a lower magnification and a larger field of vision for the shooter at close range.

I realized there was a tactical contingency for which I had not prepared. That contingency is what SWAT refers to as the "covered pile"— meaning, what if Lee had exited the lobby with a blanket over the heads of the hostages and himself? This makes target identification extremely difficult. One law enforcement agency suggested that if we had an APC near the lobby doors, it might have been feasible to stage a water cannon behind the vehicle so if the suspect exited with the hostages under a covered pile, we could use the water cannon to knock everyone down and blow away the blanket. If the device did not detonate, the snipers could differentiate targets and take appropriate action.

Another option we explored: Would a thermal device let snipers identify the heat signature of the suspect and the device? Snipers said they were not sure but did not think a thermal would help. We tested with negative results; however, newer-generation thermals may be more effective.

A good question I have been asked is why I gave the order to execute the Emergency Assault knowing that the positive block safety was not inserted. First, we could not just let three hostages die; right, wrong, or indifferent, we had to try to save them. I realized there is a lot of truth in the expression "death before dishonor." Second and most important, I had been in SWAT for twenty-six years and had done over 4,000 raids and barricades at this point, so I knew the pulse of my team. I knew they wanted to try, which was evident because as I gave the order, the two assault teams had started to move on their own initiative.

Command Lessons: One of the biggest lessons is that there is no magic "red button." In every incident, if it appears it is going to be a tactical resolution, there will be a point in time greater than all others when the likelihood of success is greatest. Command must give SWAT the opportunity to capitalize on that moment. Command cannot let a situation deteriorate and simply push the "red button" and tell SWAT to go now. Circumstances may not be suited to a favorable outcome at that point.

It is important to understand that Command has two elements feeding it information during a tactical incident: SWAT and negotiators. I say this with the utmost respect, but it is sometimes like Republican and Democrat factions, each with very strong opinions on how to resolve the incident. Each element is working hard to resolve the incident. True, negotiators resolve most incidents peacefully—always the preferred outcome that is safest for all involved. Ultimately, we are all one team, and Command is the deciding authority. While there may have been differing opinions on how to resolve the Discovery building incident, I do know the character of all the key players on that day, and all were doing what they believed to be in the best interest of the hostages and law enforcement.

Discovery Headquarters Lessons: It is also important to acknowledge the outstanding work of the Discovery headquarters management and security team. After the incident, I met with Patrick Hawk, senior director of corporate security. His team helped determine Lee's identity with law enforcement. During the incident, Hawk and his team implemented these actions:

- They quickly issued a "Do Not Admit" status to the corporate badges worn by the hostages so Lee could not use them to access other parts of the building.
- Hawk and his team maintained the camera system, providing real-time intelligence to SWAT.
- They briefed their own security and reception teams while coordinating with law enforcement.
- Corporate security implemented emergency response and evacuation plans via many communication modes: PA system, landline/cell phones, email, text message, phone bridge, radios, word of mouth.
- They assisted in evacuation of the building via an alternate exit.
- Key security and engineering personnel remained in the building to assist law enforcement.
- The communications team went to an alternate location to continue providing information.

In talking to Hawk later, I was impressed with changes his management had made three years later to improve safety for their employees. While the outcome of this incident was successful, management recognized it could do even more to enhance security and safety and so devised these changes:

- All buildings are more secure because management made structural changes.
- Discovery management redesigned the main lobby and sensory garden to better monitor people entering the lobby.
- They implemented a mass notification system.

- Employees are more aware of and versed in security procedures because Discovery management provided extra training.
- They collaborate more with law enforcement, which includes hiring armed off-duty MCPD officers to work building security.

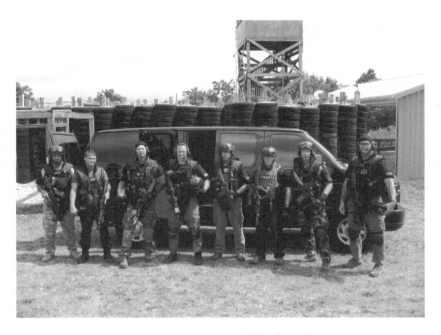

Hostage rescue training at MCPD Shoot-House
(Courtesy of MCPD)

The Discovery management was well trained and familiar with security and evacuation plans. Communications quickly began to disseminate messages and safely evacuated all employees, contractors, visitors, and children. Hawk suggested that Discovery develop a mass communication system and a backup system as well. He said it is important to plan for alternate evacuation routes/assembly areas. He pointed out that sometimes it takes an incident to remind everyone how import planning is. Discovery employees interviewed in the aftermath felt there was "nothing more that the company could have done." This statement speaks volumes.

Many factors contributed to a successful operation that day, but these are key:

- Quick, efficient response of Paden
- Discovery corporate security cooperation and pre-planning
- Efforts of Command and negotiators
- Critical intel provided by the bomb techs
- Level of training that the MCPD SWAT Team had received before the incident

Although we succeeded, I have no illusions: The outcome could have been different.

Captain Darryl McSwain, director of the Special Operations Division (SOD), and I discussed at length the courageous actions of our officers that day. We concluded that the actions of thirteen officers that day were worthy of being nominated for the department's highest award.

In nearly one-hundred years, the MCPD has bestowed only nineteen Gold Medal of Valor awards—its highest award—to recognize recipients for bravery involving extreme personal risk. Thirteen of the nineteen went to the officers who participated in the Discovery incident. Based on police officers' actions on September 1, 2010, at the Discovery building headquarters, MCPD presented Gold Medal of Valor awards to one MCPD patrol officer, eleven SWAT officers, and one member of the Montgomery County Sheriff's SRT. The SWAT officers who received the award were officers on the two Assault Teams that entered the lobby without hesitation in an effort to save the hostages. They did so with the full knowledge that the positive block safety was not inserted in the dead-man switch and that the suspect, Lee, could detonate his explosive device at any moment. Table 4 lists the awardees.

Table 4. Officers Who Received Gold Medal of Valor Awards

Name	Affiliation
Sergeant Brian Dillman	MCPD SWAT
Sergeant Brady Clouser	MCPD SWAT
Corporal Kendrick Stephens	MCPD SWAT
Officer Robert J. Kamensky	MCPD SWAT
Officer Steven Browne	MCPD SWAT
Officer Steven Phelps	MCPD SWAT
Officer Dave Reed	MCPD SWAT
Officer John McGaha	MCPD SWAT
Officer Edward Clarke	MCPD SWAT
Officer Eric Mercurio	MCPD SWAT
Officer Jordan Young	MCPD SWAT
Officer Ed Paden, Jr.	MCPD Patrol
Sheriff's Deputy Michael Stull	Montgomery County Sheriff's Department SRT

Best of the Best: Paden was the true hero of this incident. Responding "off duty," he quickly isolated the suspect, provided critical intelligence on the device via the camera system, and helped coordinate the deployment of responding officers. In 2008, Congress created the Congressional Badge of Bravery. It was created to honor local, state, and federal law enforcement officers who distinguish themselves via exceptional acts of bravery in the line of duty. Paden became the first recipient on January 9, 2012.

After the Discovery incident, I took away a critical lesson as a

SWAT commander: the significance of training. In the thirty years I spent in SWAT, I felt our team was at its highest level of preparation physically, mentally, and in terms of skill set at that moment. For the last two years before Discovery, we all had been pushing hard on training. In the seventy-two hours leading up to the Discovery incident, we had responded to two barricades and executed three raids. The team probably had about a total of six to eight hours of sleep during that entire period. The day of the Discovery incident, the team had just completed an eight-mile run. They were tired, hungry, and thirsty, yet when called upon to perform, they did so at the highest level.

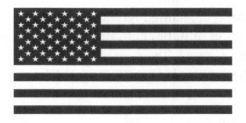

9. Diagnosis—Terminal

Uncharted

I n March of 2011, I was referred to a cardiologist at the Washington Hospital Center in DC. Once again, I underwent a vast array of testing, including rest and stress (exercise) dual-isotope scanning. I was able to reach the highest level of physical activity ever achieved in the doctor's stress laboratory. It was suggested that my ailments were age-related. I knew this was not true.

Eventually, a series of cardiac magnetic resonance imaging (MRI) scans showed enlarging wall thickness that suggested the possibility of sarcoidosis. In early August 2012, a surgeon performed a heart biopsy that came back positive for Congo red, a test that confirms a rare disease called amyloidosis. It also showed that there was extensive involvement of the heart with amyloid that contributed to my heart failure, including severe shortness of breath and swelling in the extremities.

Amyloidosis results from the accumulation of inappropriately folded proteins called amyloids. When proteins that are normally soluble in water fold to become amyloids, they become insoluble and deposit in organs or tissues, disrupting normal function. The type of protein that is misfolded and the organ or tissue in which the misfolded proteins deposit determine the clinical manifestations of amyloidosis. There are four types, each due to deposit of a specific protein. Mine was the most common type, named AL (amyloid light chain) amyloidosis, caused by deposition of light chain proteins produced by plasma cells in different disease states. The organ most affected was the heart, as evidenced by the amyloid deposits and thickening walls seen on a series of heart MRIs.

An independent bone marrow examination demonstrated 20% of plasma cells, mostly kappa restricted, which suggested I also may have a rare cancer called multiple myeloma.

Further testing produced a diagnosis of multiple myeloma cancer with cardiac AL amyloidosis.

Multiple myeloma is a cancer of plasma cells, a type of white blood cell normally responsible for providing antibodies. In multiple myeloma, collections of abnormal plasma cells accumulate in the bone marrow, where they interfere with the production of normal blood cells. Apparently, bone fractures are common with multiple myeloma because it weakens and thins the bones; hence, soon after the diagnosis, I had a skeletal survey and other bone scans done. Results showed I had a compression fracture in my back; the doctor's best estimate was that I had sustained it three years earlier. My back had hurt for a long time, but I assumed I had pulled a trapezius muscle. I iced it every night, but it never seemed to heal. I thought it had never healed due to my high work tempo.

I learned that both diseases were terminal. I had gone online and read that the average life expectancy for untreated amyloidosis was eight months. I had survived two years untreated. I also read that the average life expectancy for multiple myeloma was three to four years. There was no cure for either disease.

Mayo Clinic in Minnesota had accepted me in an effort to determine what my illness was, so the local diagnosis came just in time. I cancelled the Mayo visit and prepared for the fight of my life.

When I was diagnosed, my mom, Sandee Cropper, had been fighting ovarian cancer for two years and was in her final days. I did not want to share my diagnosis with family because I wanted them to focus on my mom. The only person who knew, other than medical staff, was Jayne.

My mother had been courageous and fought hard through her struggle with cancer. She died August 22, 2012, in Florida at the age of seventy-two. Her loving husband, Reese Cropper, Jr., had been at her side the entire two years, giving her comfort and providing her every need. I gave a eulogy at Mom's "celebration of life" on September 30, 2012, in Ocean City, Maryland. The next day, I shared my own diagnosis with my brother, Todd Offenbacher, and Mom's husband, Reese. Reese had served as president of Taylor Bank for twenty-eight years and retired with fifty-two years of service. Mom's best friend, Anna, described him as Mom's "knight in shining armor."

The following day, October 1, I advised the Command staff of the SOD, McSwain and Lieutenant Ron Smith, of my diagnosis. I advised them I was to begin chemotherapy in a week, on October 8. The treatment plan would be four to six cycles of cytoxan (chemotherapy), Velcade (a targeted chemotherapy), and dexamethasone (an anti-inflammatory steroid) that would last four to six months before doctors would consider a stem-cell transplant at the University of Maryland Medical Center (UMMC) in Baltimore. In the best-case scenario, I would be back to work doing SWAT operations in a year.

I had a huge request of the Command staff. I was retiring in two years, in October 2014. I asked to stay in SWAT in an administrative role while receiving treatment. The pride of my life is my son, Lawrence, who was ten at the time of my diagnosis. It seemed very likely that I would not survive the next two years. If I were to die, I wanted my son's last memory of his father to be that of the SWAT commander. Without hesitation, Command personnel granted my request. McSwain made a point to say, "Jeff, as long as I am in SOD, you will be here."

The MCPD SWAT Team has two SWAT supervisors (sergeants). I was the commander, and my counterpart was Dillman. This meant that the other SWAT supervisor, Dillman, would be doing double duties. He never once complained and in fact went to great lengths over the next two years to accommodate my every need. The reality was that for the next two years, Dillman was the true SWAT commander running all the operations. I was a mere puppet figure maintaining the title of commander, simply trying to survive.

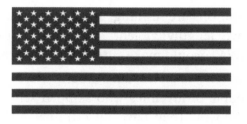

10. The Last Raid

Reflection

On October 4, 2012, I shared my diagnosis with the thirteen officers on the Central SWAT Team. The measure of support from each was overwhelming and continued for the remainder of my career. We had an early morning raid scheduled for the next day, October 5.

Every time we do a raid, we follow a definitive process to enhance the probability of success. MCPD has dozens of specialized units—Homicide, Robbery Squad, Fugitive, Special Investigations Division, District Station Investigative Section, Special Assignment Team, Firearms, Gang Unit, Auto Theft, and many more—each making on-scene arrests, generating an endless stream of search warrants and arrest warrants.

The unit that obtains a search warrant uses a threat matrix to decide if the circumstances warrant the use of SWAT: e.g., nature of the crime, criminal history of the suspect(s) or any other known occupants, weapons, and a host of other factors. We make a decision based on the totality of the information and the criteria within the matrix.

For example, detectives identify suspects wanted in residential burglaries and obtain a search warrant for a specific address where they believe the subjects are residing. The suspects have stolen multiple firearms and have lengthy violent criminal histories. Under these circumstances, SWAT would make entry and secure the suspects.

In contrast, jewelry is stolen during some daytime burglaries. The suspects are a couple of juveniles who skipped school during the day and broke into houses. They have no criminal history. Under these circumstances, the investigative unit would execute the search warrant.

Once a decision is made to use SWAT to effect entry, we assign a tactical officer to do a "drive-by." The officer designated as "security" gathers relevant information from the investigative unit and then in a covert fashion does a "drive-by," or recon, to gather further intelligence to deliver to the tactical team leader so we can develop the tactical plan.

A date, time, and staging location are set for the raid. At the staging location, investigators brief SWAT entry team personnel about significant information relevant to the raid.

The SWAT security officer then briefs the team on the operation's tactical aspects: approach, points of entry, interior layout, etc. The SWAT team leader then goes over all of the operation's finite details, individual assignments, points of entry, method of breach, and tactical contingencies.

The unit requesting SWAT assistance in serving the search warrant often sets up pre-raid surveillance on the structure. In a covert fashion, in an unmarked vehicle, personnel in plainclothes monitor the location and provide updates to SWAT and the support team. Information provided may include that the suspect vehicle is at the address, location of any lights on inside the structure, or movement observed.

When we execute the raid, we observe rules establishing areas of control for SWAT and the units supporting SWAT to follow. When SWAT approaches the location, SWAT vehicle or vehicles lead, and officers of the unit that obtained the search warrant (e.g., Robbery Squad) follow. SWAT parks at a predetermined location and quietly moves toward the suspect residence. Simultaneously, support personnel park in predetermined locations behind the SWAT vehicles and deploy quietly. The support team maintains 360-degree perimeter coverage around the structure.

The rules of responsibility are simple. SWAT controls everything in the house, and nobody enters the house until the house is cleared and SWAT declares it secure. If any subjects run from the house, SWAT does not pursue; the support perimeter element secures fleeing suspects. Specifying areas of control and responsibility avoids officers pointing firearms at each other in rapidly unfolding, dynamic situations that are often in darkness and low-light situations.

SWAT officers check everywhere in a room or area in a structure that officers have been assigned before declaring it clear—searching under clothes in a closet, lifting up couches, and searching crawl spaces and attics.

After this activity occurs and all areas appear clear and secure, two SWAT officers perform research. They go to every room and location in the structure to ensure we did not miss someone who may be hiding. We developed a research detail in the late 1980s as the consequence of a raid we did on a house occupied by gang members who had kidnapped a female and were holding her captive. During the raid, the gang members were very combative, resulting in numerous fights in the house as SWAT took suspects into custody. Several individuals leaped out of windows from second-floor bedrooms, and perimeter support personnel took them into custody. In the midst of the chaos, one gang member slipped into a closet unnoticed and hid under a pile of clothing.

We turned the structure over to investigators, believing all suspects were in custody. During the search of the premises while securing evidence related to the crime, investigators encountered the hidden suspect. Fortunately, they took the subject into custody without incident. As a result, the SWAT supervisor created a research detail in the aftermath of each raid to avoid making the same mistake again.

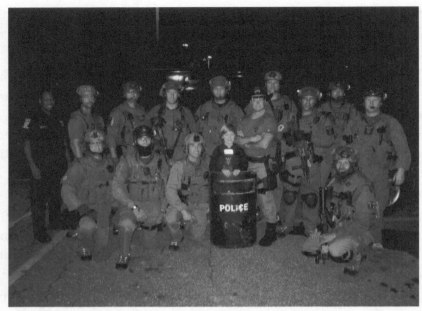

The last raid I did with the MCPD SWAT Team; my ten-year-old son, Lawrence,
accompanied me
(Courtesy of Bill Mcquiggan, MCPD)

Knowing this was likely going to be my last raid ever, I brought my son along. The team was awesome. Dillman had detailed Mcquiggan as my personal *National Geographic* photographer for the day, recognizing the significance these pictures would have to both my son and me years later. I wore a special hat during the brief. A few months earlier, team members had purchased a black Air Cavalry hat with yellow ascot, exactly like the one Robert Duvall wore in one of my favorite movies, *Apocalypse Now*. The team had a custom "T10" pin made on the front, signifying my commander's call sign, Tac 10. During the raid, my son remained outside with a tactical medic in a safe position. The medic brought him forward after the site was secure.

We had done a raid at this same location in Germantown, Maryland, four months earlier for guns and drugs, and now we were returning. We knew there were pit bulls at this location, a common ploy that drug dealers used to slow our entry. Years ago, during a raid, a pit bull bit one of our officers in the scrotum. An effective option against aggressive dogs is the deployment of a distraction device. It is much like a hand grenade, only there is no shrapnel or fragmentation. Once deployed, it has a 1.5-second delay and emits a tremendous flash and a loud bang—hence, the term "flash-bang." Ideally, we deploy it about three feet inside the door at the point of entry. Flash-bangs send any dog running and make it safer for SWAT officers, avoid officers having to shoot dogs, and allow us to reach the suspects before they retrieve weapons.

In the previous raid at this location, my assignment was to secure the kitchen. After we breached the door with the two-man battering ram, we deployed the flash-bang. I entered the kitchen and saw one of the pit bulls in the kitchen sink with his paws covering his eyes, shaking like a leaf. On the second raid, we again deployed a flash-bang with the same effect on the dogs.

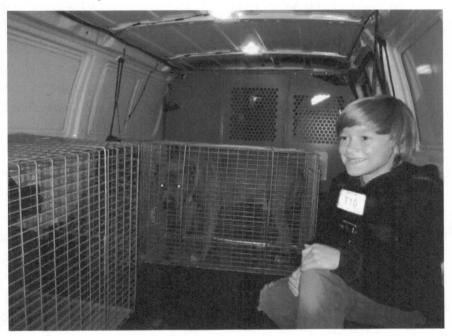

Lawrence with a caged pit bull in care of animal control after my last raid
(Courtesy of Bill Mcquiggan, MCPD)

I asked my son years later what he remembered most vividly about the raid. It was, no big surprise, the flash-bang that caused one pit bull to defecate at the front door. Officers put the front door mat over it to prevent anyone from stepping in it. Animal control took charge of the pit bulls, and the team took a picture of Lawrence sitting next to one of the caged pit bulls.

I had not yet had a chance to talk to our DSWAT officers and Sheriff's Department SRT about my diagnosis and pending treatment. After the raid I sent them the following email:

> Men, I intended to share this information personally in the near future when we were together since you are my teammates and closest friends. Unfortunately, circumstances will not allow that to occur, so I would rather you get the facts from me and put to rest any misinformation.
>
> As many of you know, my mom recently died of cancer; she was laid to rest two weeks ago.
>
> I, too, have been ill for the last two years but did not want to share that information with teammates, family, or friends because I felt the focus needed to be on getting my mom healthy. I also did not want to risk any information reaching my ten-year-old son, who was already upset about his sick grandmother.
>
> I have been diagnosed with multiple myeloma (cancer). Unfortunately, a small percentage of people with this disease also develop a secondary effect, amyloidosis, that attacks organs. In my case, the heart has been affected.
>
> There is no cure for multiple myeloma; at best, it can be put into remission, but ultimately it will return and is not survivable. The amyloidosis is more problematic than the myeloma because it has damaged my heart.
>
> Chemotherapy and other meds can place the myeloma into remission. In theory, once the myeloma is in remission, this will put the secondary effect of the amyloidosis into remission as well. The next step is a stem-cell transplant.
>
> I am starting chemotherapy and meds. In the best-case scenario, this will end just before Christmas. Then I go into the hospital for

a stem-cell transplant and will remain there for three weeks with a recovery period at home thereafter.

In a perfect world, the treatment works, and I return to work operationally in the fall. In a less-than-perfect world, there are complications, and I do not return to operations.

As of now, I am no longer operational but will still continue working as I can.

Historically, our department has made accommodations for people who are sick, injured, or have family issues. SWAT had guys out for up two years under similar circumstances. The department has afforded me the same opportunity and will allow me to stay in the unit until I recover.

If Crandell starts going through any of my gear, let me know. He will be quite embarrassed when he has to explain how a ninety-pound old man with no hair beat his ass.

No worries, just a bump in the road, because any one of us could be killed in a car crash tomorrow.

With great respect to all the men who have made this team what it is today. – Jeff

McGaha recalled that he was devastated when he read the email. He and I had a lengthy history on the team and had competed in numerous competitions together. He and I had been part of a five-man team—along with Dan Maddox, Dave Thomas, and Ray Bennett—that won the Alexandria Special Operations Team endurance competition in 1999 and 2000. Teams from the police, FBI, and the military competed. Kamensky replaced Thomas on the 2000 team. McGaha called the night I sent the email to tell me I could count on him for anything I needed. This was just the tip of the iceberg of support I got from the SWAT Team and MCPD.

On the morning of October 8, I arrived at the office of my oncologist, Dr. John Wallmark, in Rockville, Maryland, for my first chemotherapy treatment. When I walked into the reception area, the entire Central

SWAT Team, some members of the DSWAT Team, and members of the Sheriff's Department SRT were waiting. McSwain and Assistant Chief Luther Reynolds were also present, along with Jayne. I was shocked: about thirty people were present. The measure of support my team provided was overwhelming. As the nurses led me back to the fusion area, several officers and Jayne accompanied me. The limit was four guests in the treatment area.

I received a heavy dose of cytoxan, an anti-cancer drug administered intravenously and used with other medications to destroy cancer cells. I also received 20 milligrams orally of the steroid medication Dexamethasone. Finally came a shot of a targeted chemotherapy drug called Velcade (in the fatty tissue of my abdomen), classified as a proteasome inhibitor. The strategy was to put the multiple myeloma into remission and then, in theory, the amyloidosis.

Treatment occurred every Monday for three weeks straight, and then I would have one week off—a cycle. Each cycle was twenty-eight days. I would have to do at least four to six cycles before being considered for a stem-cell transplant.

I was in the fusion room for about an hour. When I came back out to the lobby, everyone was still present, providing encouragement and support. That moment spoke volumes about the relationships we had on the SWAT Team and in our police department. Dillman set up a rotation so every time I arrived for treatment, three or four SWAT officers were waiting in the lobby and stayed for the duration of my treatment. My teammates are my brothers for life.

I soon learned what effects to expect from the Monday treatments. Dexamethasone made it difficult to sleep on the first night, allowing only about two hours of rest. Wednesday and Thursdays were always my hardest days. I would be in a significant chemotherapy-induced fog that seriously impaired my cognitive abilities and made it difficult to process information. When the weekend came around, I would start to come out of the fog and feel better, with cognitive abilities improving proportionally. Then the treatment resumed for two Mondays. I greatly looked forward to the fourth week, my "off" week, as a time to recover. I would usually get about three good days out of the latter part of the fourth week. I endured the cycle to have those three good days each month. It was well worth it. Life is worth the effort.

Chemotherapy has a cumulative effect. Each week in a cycle was a little tougher than the week before. The cycles themselves also have an overall cumulative effect that wears the body down. I completed five cycles in January 2013 with little measurable benefit.

The shortness of breath was more pervasive. My legs and calves swelled to almost twice their normal size. I learned later that this was indicative of congestive heart failure. It was difficult to sleep at night because I had difficulty breathing while lying down, which is common with amyloidosis. I stacked three pillows up to breathe until it reached the point where I had to sleep upright. I purchased a pair of bed lifts that elevated the headboard by six inches, which helped tremendously. Also, my bones ached—bad. At one point, I had trouble holding my head up because my neck hurt so much. I became concerned I may need a neck brace to hold up my head.

There were a couple of nights when I thought I would not make it to morning. In the winter months, I was always cold, even though the thermostat was set at 73 degrees, so Jayne put a space heater in my room. One night stands out: I woke up about 3 a.m. and could not stop shaking. I had two blankets on the bed. I got up to put on a pair of jeans, a sweatshirt, a jacket, a knit cap, and gloves. I was feeling delirious and still could not get warm. I walked to the bathroom and dropped to my knees feeling totally exhausted. I called to Jayne, who was asleep in another room due to my snoring. She helped me to my feet and took me to my room. She grabbed her hair dryer and began blowing hot air down my sweatshirt—front and back. After about ten minutes, I started to feel better and stopped shaking. She took my temperature; it was 104. I very much felt like we had pushed the limit that night.

I talked to my brother, Todd, an avid mountain climber and adventurer. He had ample experience with the cold, having been part of a team that has led twelve adventure expeditions to the Arctic and Antarctica. He suggested that if that ever happened again, I should try some hot soup. The idea was to warm the body from the inside out.

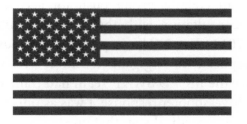

11. Stem-Cell Transplant

Fortitude

Things were not looking good when fate intervened. A good friend—John Rizak, a SWAT officer on the Arlington County Police Department in Virginia—became aware of my medical situation. Ulisney and I had trained Rizak in explosive breaching. On several occasions, we traveled to meet him in Arlington to practice our tradecraft, explosive breaching. Coincidently, Rizak was also good friends with my brother, Todd. Through a series of phone calls, Rizak learned of my grave condition. His daughter played soccer, and he had become fast friends with another parent, Dr. Richard Childs. It just so happened that Childs was a captain in the U.S. Public Health Service at the National Institutes of Health (NIH) in Bethesda, Maryland. He was responsible for the clinical research portfolio of the Division of Intramural Research at the National Heart, Lung, and Blood Institute (NHLBI) and served as a clinical policy advisor to the scientific director. The clinical research program supported more than 180 research protocols, 650 inpatient admissions, and 14,000 outpatient visits. One study focused on treatment of multiple myeloma and amyloidosis. Rizak contacted Childs and mentioned my background, including the capture of the DC snipers, and made a strong push for

NIH to accept me as a patient.

Childs made an equally strong push for acceptance, and I was scheduled for a consultation with the NIH Myeloma Branch Clinic for January 17, 2013. The NIH campus is enormous, and the high-rise building I reported to is gigantic, with several wings. Ironically, many years earlier the MCPD SWAT Team had trained the NIH Police Department in active-shooter response. I was astonished at the size and professionalism of the medical staff that greeted me on my first visit. A primary team of doctors and staff completed a comprehensive review of my medical history, diagnosis, and current treatment plan. In addition to Childs, the initial team consisted of Certified Registered Nurse Practitioner Ladan Foruraghi, Nishant Tageja, Elana Cho, and several other members.

Childs made two recommendations that had an immediate impact. First, take a specific diuretic for the fluid buildup and swelling in my lower extremities. I did so, and the vast majority of the swelling disappeared in a few days and has not recurred. Second, do not drink the green tea that I consumed daily. He noted that while there is no conclusive evidence, some researchers believe that green tea may counter the effects of some chemotherapies. I eliminated green tea and saw an improvement of my lab results upon completion of my sixth treatment cycle.

Childs is now a rear admiral (RADM: Upper) in the U.S. Public Health Service Commissioned Corps and assistant U.S. surgeon general. We've become good friends. Busy as he is, he takes time to check on my welfare. Initially, our relationship was strictly professional. As time progressed, though, we discovered that we had many common interests, including the fact that he is a major supporter of law enforcement. He enjoys shooting, has an interest in tactics, and has several firearms. He attended my retirement party, and I attended his promotional ceremony to rear admiral. I was also invited to one of his house parties. In attendance were many people from NIH who had gone to Africa with him to fight the Ebola outbreak at its peak (see photo next page). They all spoke very highly of Childs, noting that his attention to detail was one of his greatest assets.

Rizak, now retired, owns land in Middleburg, Virginia, and on occasion invites Childs for some shooting practice. On at least one occasion, Childs brought members of his team who had traveled to Africa to combat the Ebola outbreak. They shot, laughed, and ate ribs—team building at its best. I have much respect for Childs and his NIH group because they have gone to great lengths to speed me on a path to recovery.

After my preliminary visit, the NIH group consulted with a group at Tufts University in Boston, including a leading expert, Dr. Raymond Comenzo, who specializes in amyloidosis. The NIH group later obtained a second opinion from Comenzo about managing my condition; he recommended continuing the current treatment plan and proceeding posthaste to a stem-cell transplant.

One afternoon I received a phone call from Comenzo. He was on a break at a conference he was speaking at in California. He offered to take me as a patient and perform the stem-cell transplant.

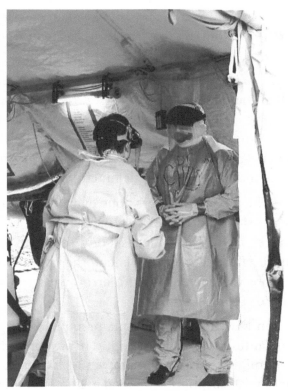

Certainly, having the best was a very appealing offer. The fact that he took the time to make the call himself spoke volumes about his dedication to his profession. As it turned out, though, Dr. Ashraf Z. Badros at UMMC was already evaluating me for an autologous stem-cell transplant. He

Dr. Richard Childs in a biohazard suit in Africa with his Ebola team at the height of the crisis

(Courtesy of NIH)

had extensive clinical experience with bone marrow transplantation and a special interest in multiple myeloma. Ultimately, I declined Comenzo's offer for several reasons. I would have had to make multiple trips to Boston for the prep phase, the transplant, and post exams. I wanted to be close to my son, Jayne, my family, and the SWAT Team.

The NIH group, Wallmark, and Badros, who would perform the transplant, all continued consulting Comenzo, who even today remains a valuable resource.

I was very fortunate to have a group of extremely knowledgeable doctors from an assortment of medical groups comparing notes and collectively deciding the best course of action.

UMMC performed pre-transplant tests to evaluate my health and determine if a transplant would be safe and appropriate. An NIH MRI team also did a cardiac risk assessment of a stem-cell transplant because of the amyloid in the heart. I was cleared through both sets of tests.

In an autologous transplant, the medical staff removes and reserves some of the patient's own bone marrow or peripheral blood stem cells. Then the patient receives high doses of chemotherapy or radiation to destroy cancer cells. Afterward, the staff reinfuses the patient's blood cells through a transfusion. These cells find their way to the bone marrow and begin producing new blood cells. Through this process, the patient's bone marrow and immune functioning return to normal.

The procedure offers hope of an extended remission or even a cure when standard cancer treatment has not been able to destroy all the cancer cells. The patient's body can withstand higher and possibly more effective doses of chemotherapy and/or radiation, which can restore the current bone marrow function with fresh bone marrow and/or stem cells.

In March 2013, I began a prep phase for a transplant that involved implanting a chemotherapy port in my upper chest below the collar bone. It administered chemotherapy and facilitated drug administration for optimal absorption and blood extraction for lab evaluations. On March 22, I received a heavy infusion of cytoxan chemotherapy at UMMC. I had to self-administer Neupogen injections to the abdomen daily for ten days straight. Jayne became my self-administrator. The Neupogen mobilized stem cells from the bone marrow into the bloodstream.

On April 2, I reported to UMMC for stem-cell collection. The medical team processed, froze, and stored the stem cells until the day of the transplantation.

On April 10, I was told to report to a conference room at police headquarters for a discussion of active-shooter protocols. When I walked into the room, my son was present, along with all of the Central and DSWAT Team.

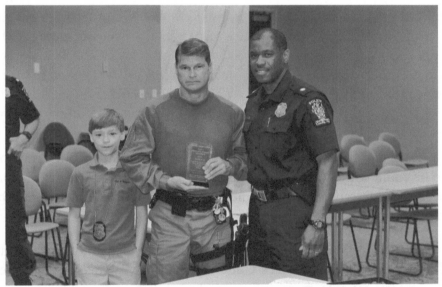

Receiving the Living Legend Award from Assistant Chiefs Darryl McSwain and Luther Reynolds (April 2013)
(Courtesy of MCPD)

McSwain, Reynolds, and other executive officers were also present. McSwain and Reynolds called me forward to receive the Living Legend Award. The engraving read:

Living Legend Award, presented to Sergeant Lawrence "Jeff" Nyce, April 10, 2013. In appreciation for extraordinary service and commitment to excellence over the past thirty-two years. You are an outstanding example to all of us. SOD MCPD.

I had known McSwain for many years. Eventually, he achieved the rank of assistant chief in our department and moved on to become chief of police in the Maryland-National Capital Park Police's Montgomery County Division. He and I have always been very good friends. He is physically fit so we sometimes worked out together, and I helped design workout programs for him. We both have an interest in military history, and on occasion he has been to my house to watch movies or have dinner. Our paths still cross as we frequent police functions.

Likewise, I have known Reynolds for many years and become friends with him. He went on to become chief of police; in his case, it was the city of Charleston, South Carolina. He was the person who gave me the opportunity to become the SWAT commander at MCPD. We worked out together occasionally and took our sons on white-water rafting expeditions in Harpers Ferry, West Virginia. Reynolds was familiar with Harpers Ferry because he attended one of the team-building days we hosted there for the Central and DSWAT Teams.

I was dumbfounded but extremely grateful that they brought my son so he could witness the event. The timing of the event—five days before my stem-cell transplant—gave me renewed strength as I moved into the unknown.

On April 15, I arrived at the hospital. The transplant unit, on the ninth floor of the medical center's Gudelsky Building, is specially designed to protect patients from infection during recovery. After receiving chemotherapy and/or radiation, a patient's white blood cell count is low. Since we need white blood cells to fight infection, the hospital cleans the air in each room continuously using a high-efficiency particulate air, or HEPA, filter. A dedicated team of experienced doctors and nurses trained in cancer and transplant cared for me. They taught me and my family what we needed to know about care and recovery.

My room was small, with a bathroom. I had a great view of Baltimore. When I looked out at the ten o'clock position (slightly to the left), I could see the Orioles' stadium about a mile away. At the two o'clock position (right), was the Ravens' stadium about a mile and a half away.

The day I checked into the hospital, the Boston Marathon bombings occurred, killing three people and wounding 287. The city was on lockdown as police searched for the suspects. I thought: "How fortunate I was that I chose to have my stem-cell transplant in Baltimore instead of Boston." I wondered how that event, with a massive number of casualties, would have affected my treatment had I selected Boston.

The SWAT Team assisted Jayne in bringing the items I would need for the next three weeks. They smuggled in some lightweight dumbbells (ten to twenty-five pounds) in a duffle bag. I decided no matter how bad I felt, I would try to do some light weights and walk on one of the treadmills in the exercise room each day ("a body at rest stays at rest, and a body in motion stays in motion"). I knew it was important to be active at some level.

Early on, since my first chemo treatment, I developed a strategy for survival. Cancer is aggressive, so I needed to be equally aggressive. I strongly felt that the fact that I had been in good physical condition had contributed to me still being alive. I also realized that my energy pool had diminished a lot. Cancer and the medications to treat it cause fatigue. Recognizing the reduced energy levels, I decided there were two things I would do every day. First, make my bed to give me a sense of accomplishment at the start of the day. It also gave me a sense of order during a very disordered phase of my life. Second, work out, no matter how poorly I felt.

Each day when I woke up, I felt nauseous and dizzy and had a headache. I soon discovered that if I could sustain thirty minutes of physical activity, my head would clear, and I would start to feel better. I wondered if it was the positive effect of the endorphins that release as a result of exercise. Continuing physical exercise for the first thirty minutes proved to be difficult.

My shortness of breath and swelling of the lower extremities had become so bad before using diuretics that I could no longer run. I started swimming, hoping my legs would not swell as much. It took all my effort to complete one lap. I would stop after each lap and put my head in my arms on the deck while standing in the lane. I would rest for one to two minutes, completely out of breath, regroup, and swim another lap. I would do from twenty-six to one-hundred laps (on one occasion), depending on how I felt. The swims took a long time to complete, but at least I was doing something aerobic at whatever level I could.

I went to the gym to lift weights as well. I would only focus on one repetition at a time and then try to do just one more rep. I needed about five minutes of rest between sets. I would regroup and then hit another set. It was critical to continue resistance training to keep my bones strong given the multiple myeloma. I spent much of my day just getting through these workouts that drained my daily pool of energy. Often after dinner, I would put my head in my hands, completely exhausted and in a daze; it was not uncommon that I would be asleep by 7:30 p.m.

I didn't realize it, but I had learned a lot watching my mother's fight with cancer. First, there were occasions when she had a gap in treatment. Each time there was a gap, her condition deteriorated. Gaps in treatment can occur for many reasons. Sometimes they are needed because lab results are not within the norm, and it would be unsafe to administer treatment. Some patients need a break because they can no longer tolerate the treatment.

I was determined not to have a gap in treatment. Wallmark has an online system that lets patients access all their laboratory and test results—a great resource because I could track the progress of my treatment *and* determine how diet and nutrition can influence lab results.

Because I was dealing with numerous challenging test results and side effects, I began doing research on nutritional alternatives to return my lab results and condition to normal/safe ranges. Table 5 reflects the impact of nutritional changes on my lab results.

Table 5. Corrective Actions to Counter Medical Challenges

Challenge Type	Corrective Action	Outcomes	Timeframe
Low white blood cell count	Lentils and kiwi	Returned to normal for 8 years	3-4 weeks
Low platelet count	Omega-3 fats—salmon daily	Returned to normal	2 weeks
Liver: High alkaline phosphatase (ALP), alanine aminotransferase (ALT), aspartate aminotransferase (AST)	Water and lemon juice	Returned to normal	2 weeks
High kidney creatinine level	• Berry fruits: blackberry, blueberry, raspberry, strawberry • Hydration—water quarts daily	Returned to normal	4 weeks
Inflammation	Turmeric with black pepper	Reduced inflammation	2 weeks
Constipation	Fibrous food daily and laxatives	Normal bowel movement	2 weeks
Low potassium—caused severe cramping	• Potassium supplement • Hydration—water quarts daily	Significant reduction	1 week

Preparation is the key to success in any pursuit—whether it be studying for an exam, being successful in business, competing in an athletic event, or preparing for a SWAT operation. I took my nutritional lessons learned and developed a plan for success. I am an early riser, waking up around 5:30 a.m. I fast every day for at least twelve hours (more in Chapter 16). Table 6 indicates the diet that has helped me remain in remission for two years.

Table 6. Cancer-Sensitive Diet

Meal	Food	Benefit

Breakfast	• Scrambled together:
	  ○ Three egg whites
	  ○ One full egg with yolk
	  ○ Shitake mushrooms
	  ○ Garlic
	• Seasoned with turmeric and black pepper
	  ○ Lentils
	  ○ Lemon juice and water
		• High protein, low fat
		
		• Anti-inflammatory
		
		• High white blood cell count; low-calorie carb
		• Liver function—ALT, ALP; stabilizes glucose levels

Lunch	• Turkey sandwich with avocado topping • Lemon juice and water	• Omega-3 for platelet count; high protein/ low calorie • Liver function—ALT, AST, ALP
Dinner	• Grilled chicken or salmon • Fibrous vegetable • Lemon juice and water	• Omega-3 for platelet count; high protein/ low calorie • Good bowel movement • Liver function—ALT, AST, ALP; stabilizes glucose
Snacks (2-3)	Plain Greek yogurt; fresh berries	Lowers creatinine level—kidney function

Close friend Drew Tracy, who survived stage 4 throat cancer, had some outstanding advice. He was my SWAT sergeant early in my career and had won the "toughest cop alive competition" years ago. A fighter by nature, he said, "Don't read the Internet because it will only tell you that you are going to die." He also said, "You have to be your own advocate when it comes to your treatment." His words proved to be very true. I had been browsing the Internet and, in essence, felt as though I had received a death sentence. While I intended to fight the cancer, I did look at cemeteries, and I drew up a living will.

I believe that life is all about perspective. Every man is his own legacy, and it matters not what happened to those before me. I decided that someone had to survive these diseases. I told my doctors that I would be the person to survive. If I never stopped believing, I could accomplish anything. Faced with this prognosis, I had a choice: Wait to die or choose to live. I chose to live.

My life has turned into a lengthy series of challenges, similar to navigating an obstacle course. I had been diagnosed with multiple myeloma and amyloidosis. Then my treatment went from four chemo cycles to six. A prep phase for a stem-cell transplant and hospitalization followed. I would need to survive a lengthy, exhausting recovery period that would utterly deplete my strength. Then more chemotherapy would be necessary for the rest of my life, constantly depleting energy and strength.

Initially, the experience seemed overwhelming. I surmounted all challenges by attacking them as I would an obstacle course. I focused on nothing but the obstacle directly before me and hit each as aggressively as I could. Once I cleared one obstacle, I regrouped en route to the next and hit it as aggressively as possible, repeating the technique over and over until I completed the course.

Despite the constant challenges I was to confront, I still felt fortunate. I had lived a full life and had the opportunity to serve on one of the finest police departments in the nation. My illness hit me late in my career, and I would have a pension to fall back on. I recognized I had the full support of the department, family, and friends. Their extraordinary measure of support overwhelmed me and made me realize that sometimes we forget just how blessed we are.

I am not particularly religious and rarely go to church, but I have always believed strongly in the Lord Jesus Christ. Each morning I say the same prayer: "Lord Jesus Christ and guardian angel (Mom), thank you for another day on this Earth. You are the guiding light in my life and the savior of my soul. With you I am everything; without you I am nothing. Thank you, Lord Jesus Christ and guardian angel, for all you do for me and all of mankind. I love you both for it. Mom, I miss you and love you. Lord Jesus Christ and guardian angel, have a great day. Give me great strength to get through another day. Amen."

Another factor in my survival is devotion to my son, Lawrence. I wanted to watch him grow to be a man and provide him guidance. I wanted to share in his early achievements—getting his driver's license, getting his first job, and graduating from high school.

Thirty years in SWAT prepared me for this fight. There were three things that I always expected from the men in SWAT: Never complain, never quit, and the mission comes first. Failure's not an option as it relates to the mission. The men with whom I worked always delivered on these expectations. I applied the same expectations to myself in this situation: Never complain, never quit, and the mission comes first. The mission is survival, and failure's not an option.

I was getting settled into my room at the transplant unit when Badros came by to educate me about the procedure and what would occur. Today, he said, I would receive 140 mg of the chemotherapy melphalan, a reduced dose because the amyloid in my heart made higher doses too risky. He said there is a 5% chance of death associated with this procedure. I asked him what the highest dose is a patient can receive. He said, under ideal circumstances, 200 mg. I said I wanted to receive the highest dose and the full benefits of a stem-cell transplant.

He said: "No; it's too risky."

I explained that my entire life had been about pushing the limit and that I accepted the higher risk because I knew I was dying, and this was my one chance at life. He re-emphasized that 200 mg would significantly increase the risk.

I said: "I accept the risk." And I told him: "I promise I will not die."

Reluctantly, he agreed to the 200 mg dose. I thanked him.

Two days later, on April 17, I received my stem-cell transplant. Jayne, who is also an MCPD officer, was working half days and driving to the hospital. Visiting hours were restricted so they did not start until afternoon. Badros was present along with a team of medical support staff. The peripheral stem cells that the staff had frozen and processed were brought to my room in the transplant unit. The cells thawed at my bedside in a warm solution. The staff administered them via an IV line attached to my port. They said I may experience a funny taste in my mouth and an odd smell during the procedure that may last up to forty-eight hours—due to the preservative dimethyl sulfoxide being used in the freezing process. They also advised me that I may experience side effects such as nausea, shortness of breath, stomach cramping, and wheezing. The infusion takes about sixty minutes. Afterward, I would receive medications/antibiotics to prevent infection, nausea, or vomiting.

I had been told I had two and a half bags of stem cells to process. They appeared to be in clear IV bags. When one bag was empty, staff replaced it with another bag until the process was complete.

The transplant began. It was not painful, but after the first bag, I started to feel loopy—very loopy. The staff asked if I was okay. I said I was, even though I felt as if things were going south. I knew this was my one-time shot at life, and I needed to get all the stem cells in me. I did not want to say anything that would end the procedure. I remember the second bag being switched out and the staff asking again if I was okay. I said I was, and soon thereafter, I began to have an out-of-body experience, flying with my arms out like a bird soaring high over the city of Baltimore. I flew over the hospital and flew lower. From above, I peered through the window of my room and could see myself lying in bed receiving the transplant. I suddenly snapped out of it, returned to my bedside, and saw the final drops empty from the last IV bag.

The next thing I recall was waking up with a large number of medical staff present. To the left of my bed, I saw two technicians with the electric shock pads of a defibrillator on a crash cart. Apparently, my blood pressure dropped significantly, and I lost consciousness. I became unresponsive and coded just after the last stem cells were transplanted. Chest compressions and intravenous saline brought me back.

The medical team was arranging to transfer me immediately to the intensive care unit (ICU). While awaiting transfer, I called Jayne and then Dillman. Jayne recalls the conversation. I said: "I coded, and I have to go." She said, "What?" and I hung up. Jayne tried to call me back, but I did not pick up. She said she started shaking and immediately called the hospital nurses in the transplant wing. The nurses advised her I was okay, and Jayne proceeded immediately to the hospital. When she arrived, I was still in the transplant wing waiting for the transfer to ICU. Two technicians were standing by my door with equipment in case I had another medical emergency before reaching ICU.

Dillman was at the outdoor firearms range with the team when I called him.

I told him: "I am not sure what happened, but I think I coded, and I am being transferred to ICU."

He asked: "What do you need me to do?"

"Nothing," I said. "Thanks."

After the staff stabilized me, I spent the night in ICU and was released to the transplant unit the following day. Badros came to my room.

He said: "I knew I shouldn't have given you 200 mg," referring to the melphalan chemotherapy.

I could see he was upset. I told him, "Dr. Badros, you did exactly what I asked you to do. I am glad you did because I now have a real chance at survival."

I admired the man for having the courage and strength to think outside the box. I am sure that there are medical professionals who would say he shouldn't have done it. I firmly believe that I would not be alive today if he had not administered the 200 mg of melphalan chemotherapy that is the standard dosage for best clinical results.

Dying at that moment seemed pale compared to the suffering and pain I had endured for the previous six months. Now I just faded out; there was no pain.

Back in the transplant unit, I had some special attire that I had brought to wear that day.

I put on my black Air Cavalry hat with yellow ascot, just like Robert Duvall in the classic beach scene in *Apocalypse Now*.

Duvall played Lieutenant Colonel Bill Kilgore, whose unit had just captured a Viet Cong village during the Vietnam war. Kilgore ordered a napalm strike by fighter jets that ended the battle. He then kneeled down on one knee, picked up some sand in one hand, and said to some of his men: "I love the smell of napalm in the morning. You know, one time we had a hill bombed for twelve hours. When it was all over, I walked up. We didn't find one of 'em, not one stinkin' body. The smell, you know that gasoline smell, the whole hill. Smelled like victory."

I knelt down as Duvall did. Jayne took a picture on my cell phone. I sent the photo out to the SWAT Team with a caption, "I love the smell of stem cells in the morning; smells like victory."

The transplant unit imposed a number of safety precautions. Visitor hours were from noon until 10:00 p.m., with only two visitors at a time in the room. Because of the risk of infection, visitors had to be at least twelve years of age. Visitors must wash their hands before entering the room and may not use the patient's bathroom. Plants and flowers were not permitted. I was free to leave my room and roam the transplant unit. Any time I left my room, I had to wear a protective mask.

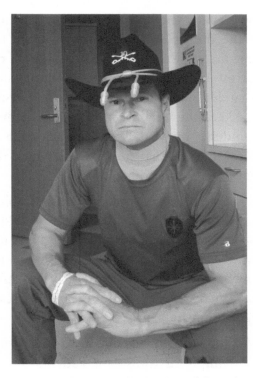

There was a lounge area at the far end of the unit with couches—a place to read or for family and friends to visit. It also had several treadmills and exercise bikes. Staff encouraged light exercise.

Since I had coded during the transplant, staff watched me closely. I had a mobile medical pole cart next to my bed with many lines and tubes so they could

The day after my stem-cell transplant: "I love the smell of stem cells in the morning; smells like victory"

(Courtesy of Jayne Nyce, MCPD)

monitor my vitals constantly.

I had done a light workout every day since admission and was determined to continue to do so. I had trained the morning of the day I coded. The day I was released from ICU, I had not yet worked out. I thought: "Day One, post-transplant; let's do this."

I felt weak and nauseous and had a headache. I put on my protective mask, exited my room, wheeled my cart to the exercise room, and started walking on the treadmill at an incredibly slow pace. Every step was an effort. After about five to ten minutes, a group of nurses rushed into the exercise room, explaining that I needed to notify them when I left the room to exercise. Apparently, my heart rate increased significantly with the walking, and the heart monitors alerted the staff to a potential medical problem. There was no problem—just the result of light exercise.

After completing my twenty-minute walk, I returned to my room. I now got out the light dumbbells that the team had smuggled in for me. The only place with enough space to train was the bathroom. Unfortunately, this again caused my heart rate to rise. The nurses knew I was not on the treadmill, so a medical team responded and caught me red-handed with the weights. They were all really good about it: they let me keep the weights, so I notified them any time I exercised for the remainder of my visit. It was actually quite comforting to know that the medical staff was that attentive and would respond at a moment's notice if they perceived a problem.

Post-stem-cell transplant is a miserable existence. My white blood cell count was extremely low. I was told it would eventually reach zero—a normal part of the recovery. I was incredibly weak and fatigued. I always felt nauseous and had a perpetual headache. I developed a rash on my back and neck on about Day Two after the transplant. A team of specialists responded, did numerous tests, treated it, and the rash went away after several days.

All food tasted metallic as they said it would. Despite this, I still got cravings. All transplant patients have a nutritionist assigned to administer a special diet. The hospital provided meals. Jayne visited almost every day, one day bringing some homemade tuna fish salad I wanted. It looked great, but when I took a couple of bites, it tasted like metal. Staff told me that my sense of taste would return after several months. Despite food not tasting good, I never lost my appetite.

Early on, I did not want any visitors other than Jayne. I was always so tired. After she had driven an hour to visit me, I usually fell asleep within forty-five minutes of her arrival. Then she would then drive home. I probably slept sixteen hours a day.

My dad, Larry Nyce, and his wife, Jane, visited several times. He had retired from American University after thirty years as a professor of physical education and tennis coach. He was a good father, and his discipline greatly contributed to my sense of responsibility. Karl Offenbacher, my brother's father, and his wife, Alpana, visited. Karl was a successful businessman who owned Offenbacher Pool and Patio. It was great having the support.

On April 25, eight days after the transplant, my white blood cell count reached zero. I had never before been so fatigued and weak. I tried to sleep as much as I could. A person is never more acutely aware that he is alive than when he is suffering greatly. When blood counts are very low, engraftment occurs: The infused bone marrow or peripheral blood stem cells "take" and begin producing blood cells. It may take ten to sixteen days for engraftment to occur.

Despite the way I felt, I still managed to walk and lift weights daily. When I was first faced with the prospect of being in a hospital for three weeks, I asked myself what I could do to occupy myself. I had brought books, and there were projects I wanted to complete on my laptop. I didn't read one book or complete one project. It was too difficult to stay focused, and I slept most of the time.

The SWAT guys had wanted to visit on the day of the transplant, but I nixed that idea. When I felt better, they visited and made me laugh. We told stories and carried on for about an hour in the lounge. It was great to see them.

Finally, on May 1, I was discharged. Jayne, who was assigned as my primary caretaker, had to take a class on follow-up care. She was very attentive and took notes.

Some SWAT guys assisted in loading my vehicle. It felt great to leave the hospital. The doctors and nurses had all been outstanding. I was grateful to have had such a professional group.

It was important that I obey a set of safety rules designed to minimize the risk of complications. I would be extremely susceptible to infection for the next ninety days. Jayne had the carpet at her house steam cleaned. Anytime I left the house, I still had to wear a protective mask that was disposable and for one-time use only. I was to avoid animals and small children. All meals had to be made at home—no outside or restaurant food. All meats had to be cooked to a temperature over 165 degrees. I was not permitted to eat leftovers. All vegetables, fruits, and salads had to be thoroughly washed. There were lots of food rules.

Jayne is into fitness, understands my rules, and has always been good about preparing healthy meals. I kid her that she was a doctor in her previous life because she has an acute interest in the medical profession. She is facile at treating ailments and injuries I have sustained over the years—caretaker par excellence! Fortunately, she can live any desire she has to be a doctor vicariously through her son, Brett Bowers, a doctor of optometry.

Life post-transplant was going to require adjusting to a strict health regimen.

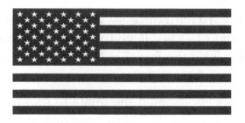

12. Fooling the Trained Observers

Perception

I was now back at home at last, but I faced a long haul in recovering over the next ninety days. To deal with the boredom of serious restrictions needed to prevent complications, I decided to seek some entertainment. The escapade started two weeks after my liberation from the hospital when Todd flew in from Lake Tahoe. He had sent me a picture of himself indicating that he had shaved his head to honor me. I told him: "Big thanks, but I have not lost any hair, and sorry, but I am not shaving it for you." We laughed.

His shaved head gave me an idea for a practical joke. The day before Todd arrived, a teammate named Jordan Young gave me a ride to a follow-up visit with Badros, a fact that eventually played a role in my scheme. In all the years I had been in SWAT, I had never been able to pull off a practical joke. The guys could just read right through me. I told Young that my brother, whose head was shaved, was coming to town. We are of similar height, weight, and build, so I suggested that he tell the team that during my visit with Badros, I lost all my hair.

During my illness, the team would typically invite me to join them at Panera for breakfast after they went on an early morning raid. They would always want to eat before an early morning workout. When I was healthy, I was adamant that I wanted to work out first and eat later, so I usually gave them a hard time, saying: "You haven't worked out yet, so you haven't earned the privilege to eat." They would all laugh and take issue with me about the fact that I was more interested in exercise than food.

Even so, I always appreciated the invite to join the team, especially after I got sick. The plan that day in the summer of 2013 was to join the team at breakfast after a raid. I would send my brother in with his shaved head, dressed in a pair of blue jeans, black sweatshirt with our SWAT emblem, and black Salomon hiking shoes, which is what I typically wore when off duty. He would wear a protective mask covering half his face and so look like me.

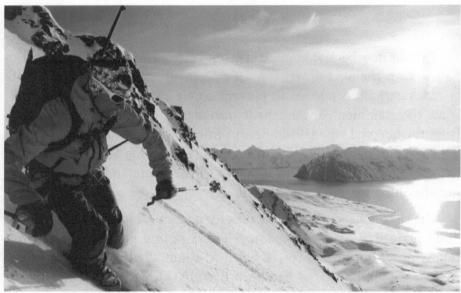

Adventure guide Todd skiing in the Arctic Circle, living the dream
(Courtesy of Court Leve)

Aside from being an avid mountain climber/adventurer, Todd was then and remains host of a TV morning show in Lake Tahoe. Despite our similar looks, my brother is everything I am not. I am very serious;

he is comical, funny, and a practical joker by nature, so this stunt was right up his alley. He has also been a competitive bodybuilder, finishing as the runner-up in the 1981 Teen Mr. America and second in the 1985 Mr. USA AAU medium class as an adult. He was in the music video for the song "Muscles" by Diana Ross in 1982. Todd was co-owner of a gym called Aeroflex in the 1990s in Rockville, Maryland. He moved to California to pursue his interests as an adventurer and a thrill seeker, a role that eventually landed him a job working for a company named Outside TV as a morning-show host in Lake Tahoe.

Several days after he arrived, we met the team for breakfast. I pulled into the Panera parking lot and recognized our unmarked tactical SWAT vehicles.

I sent Todd in first. He knew my idiosyncrasies, habits, and catchphrases.

Other than Jordan, the team had not seen me since I had left the hospital, so they had no sense of what I might look like.

Todd walked to the rear of the restaurant where the team typically sat. The team saw him, and guys called out, "Hey, Sarge!" Stephens, seated, invited Todd to sit across from him and asked him about an email that he had sent.

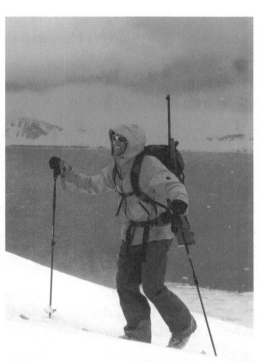

Brother Todd ski guiding in Svalbard in the Arctic Circle (3,000 hungry polar bears) with rifle
(Courtesy of Court Leve)

Todd kept his head low and muttered one of my catchphrases:

"Roger that."

Browne asked: "Can I get you a cup of coffee?"

Todd, with his head low, muttered: "Yes, can I get a sesame bagel also?"

Todd later told me he knew he was pushing the limit, but he was also hungry.

Browne bought a cup of coffee and a bagel for Todd.

When another teammate asked Todd a question, he responded with another one of my catchphrases: "Yippee-ki-yay."

The entire time, Todd kept his head and voice low and portrayed an ill individual.

After about five minutes, I came in with a full head of hair, dressed identically to Todd. I walked over to the team and said, "I see you met my brother, Todd."

For a brief moment, you could have heard a pin drop. Browne then said, looking at Todd: "You bastard, I bought you a cup of coffee!"

Dillman and Tatakis said: "It is a good thing you came in when you did." Tatakis had always looked after my welfare, so I referred to him as the Spartan because of his Greek origins. Todd was so convincing and appeared so sick they were getting ready to call an ambulance to take him to Shady Grove Medical Center for a checkup.

We all laughed. Finally, after thirty-two years, I pulled off a practical joke. Actually, Todd did the job. He told me later he was hoping these guys had a sense of humor, or he would have been in serious trouble.

I continued wearing the protective mask every time I left the house. My sense of taste came back after about two months. Jayne is a phenomenal cook and good about attending to my dietary needs. I could finally enjoy her meals. I looked forward to the day the mask would come off so I could eat out at a nice restaurant.

After my stem-cell transplant and during my recovery period, my good friend Steve Lockshin visited and did some remarkable things for me. I met him through my brother because both had gone to Wootton High School.

Our friendship grew when my brother opened Aeroflex gym in Rockville, Maryland. Todd had served as Lockshin's personal trainer for many years, and when my brother moved to Lake Tahoe, I took over as his fitness consultant. We worked out together for years, and he excelled physically.

Lockshin is an incredibly successful and gracious individual: founder and former CEO of Convergent Wealth Advisors, one of the nation's leading wealth management firms, which provides investors with objective advice and flexible investment solutions. He is also a founder and principal of AdvicePeriod. He is a well-recognized entrepreneur in the investment community and is the author of a book titled *Get Wise to Your Advisor.*

There was a ring at the doorbell, and Lockshin knew that after my stem-cell transplant I spent the vast majority of my day isolated in bed rest. Two workers delivered a brand-new Samsung 55-inch flat-screen TV. They came in, mounted it on a wall in my bedroom, and said: "This is courtesy of Steve Lockshin; he will stop by later today."

That is the kind of guy he is. On April 1, 2002, the Maryland Terrapins men's basketball team played for the NCAA National Championship against the Indiana Hoosiers at the Georgia Dome in Atlanta, Georgia. Lockshin knew I was a huge Maryland basketball fan, and he called me on Sunday, the day before the game. He said: "If I can get tickets, do want to go?" I said: "Are you kidding me? Of course." He said he would get back to me later in the day, and while that would have been a dream come true, I had no expectation that it would occur. Several hours later, he called and said to be at a particular location at Dulles International Airport at 10:00 the next morning. When I arrived, his plane and a second plane were waiting.

Lockshin owned a Pilatus PC-12 single-engine turboprop passenger aircraft. The cabin area was spacious, with large windows and reclining leather seats. It had a cruising speed of 311 mph and a maximum altitude of 30,000 feet and was equipped with the latest avionics. I believe it could hold ten passengers plus the pilot. Lockshin was also a pilot, working hard to earn his various certifications and licenses. More than a dozen of us split up between the two aircraft, and when we landed in Atlanta, there were two limos waiting. Lockshin took us to dinner and then the Georgia Dome, where I watched the Maryland Terrapins win their first national championship, 64-52. After the game, a limo took us to the airport, and we flew back home. Turnaround time was less than twenty-four hours, absolutely amazing. While this lifestyle may have been the norm for Lockshin and his business associates, as a simple cop, I was dumbfounded. I saved my ticket for memory's sake, but unfortunately, I misplaced it when I moved.

In September of 2013, Lockshin once again performed one of his many kind acts. He owned a yacht that was berthed at San Juan Island, just north of Seattle. He invited my brother, his family, Jayne, and me to stay on his boat. Reese flew out and joined us. The boat was a luxurious Sunseeker Manhattan yacht, named *B-Yacht'ch*. It could sleep all of us, and Lockshin offered its use. It was an incredible trip. We took a seaplane from Seattle to San Juan Island. This was the first traveling I had done since my stem-cell transplant. One day, we hired a captain whom Lockshin had recommended to take us out to sea. We saw more than a dozen orcas, and it felt great to get out on the open sea and feel the fresh air after having been isolated in a hospital and a bedroom for so long. It was a unique adventure for me. I had never been on a seaplane, never slept overnight on a yacht, and never seen orcas. Best of all, I shared all these experiences with family.

To this day, Lockshin calls and checks on my welfare.

I slept a great deal the first year after the stem-cell transplant. I had been told by the doctors I could expect to go back to work six to twelve months after the transplant. I continued to work out

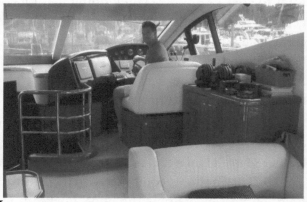

Lockshin's yacht, named B-Yacht'ch; note the dumbbells he purchased for my use (right side)

(Courtesy of Jayne Nyce)

each day, and after six weeks, I decided to go back to work. I would go in for about four hours a day and do what I could. I didn't have to work; I had accumulated enough leave to take off until I retired. I just loved the job at any level.

We had a new Command staff at SOD that included Captain Bob Bolesta, Lieutenant Eric Stancliff, and Lieutenant Frank Stone. They gave me great latitude, letting me come and go as I needed. Some days were better than others. It was important to regain some sense of normality. Being around a supportive Command staff and seeing the team greatly lifted my spirits.

The ninety-day mark arrived, the mask came off, and Jayne and I went out to dinner. At the one-hundred-day mark, I had a bone marrow biopsy that would indicate whether the transplant had succeeded. The transplant achieved positive results, but I did not reach remission. More high-dose chemotherapy treatment would be required to attempt to achieve remission. I restarted cycles of chemotherapy with Velcade, Revlimed, and dexamethasone.

Drew Tracy, now an assistant chief, called one day wanting to meet for lunch. He has always looked after me. We met at a restaurant in Gaithersburg. He led us to a table in the back of the restaurant. Seated at the table were Keith Runk from the MSP and Chuck Pierce, William T. McCarthy, Paul T. Jaskot, and Neil Darnell from the FBI. These were the guys on the DC snipers Assault Team. Tracy knew I was still struggling with my health and so gathered the group for a reunion. It was great seeing all these guys as we reminisced. I think Tracy knew that it was questionable as to how much longer I was going to be around. Seeing these guys offer so much support gave me great strength and reinforced my will to survive.

After about four months, I was able to do an eight-hour day at work. Since I could no longer do raids as an operator, the Command staff let me respond to ERT callouts/barricades, etc., and provide tactical input on the Command bus. In January of 2014, there was an active-shooter incident at Columbia Mall in Howard County. Howard County SWAT reached out to multiple outside agencies for help. Our agency responded, and I did as well to assist our Command staff.

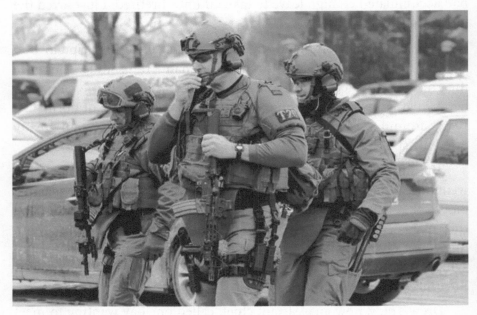

MCPD SWAT after responding to an active shooter at Columbia Mall in January 2014; three
dead including the suspect (in support of Howard County SWAT)
(Courtesy of MCPD)

The heavy doses of chemotherapy again left me in a mental fog that
I noticed during this callout, so after the incident, I told Command
personnel that I would no longer respond to ERT callouts. I felt the
chemotherapy made decision-making and processing information too
difficult. It was important for me to recognize my limitations.

When I was first diagnosed in 2012, I knew my career in SWAT was
over and set a retirement date of October 1, 2014.

I was still in serious discomfort, and every day felt like a struggle to
stay alive. I truly did not know if I would make it to my retirement. Then,
suddenly, in May 2014, I started to feel much better and stronger.

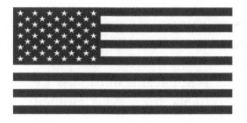

13. SWAT Selection Standards

Mindset

I am often asked: "What does it take to become a SWAT officer?" Standards vary from state to state and jurisdiction to jurisdiction. In Montgomery County, Maryland, we have a defined process. As noted earlier, we maintain two SWAT Teams. A full-time team does nothing but SWAT operations. The current full-time team has two supervisors (sergeants) and fifteen officers. The DSWAT Team has part-time officers who are assigned to other department units, are trained in SWAT tactics, and supplement the full-time team as needed. The DSWAT Team has seventeen officers from the rank of sergeant down.

MCPD has 1,200 officers. The Central Team constitutes 1% of the total force, and the Central and Decentralized Teams between them constitute just 3% of the total force.

When vacancies occur on the Central Team, we fill them with a DSWAT member. The DSWAT Team is a grooming process. Typically, we select the more senior DSWAT officers based on training, experience, and observation of their job performance in an operational environment.

When we fill vacancies on the Central Team, this creates a shortage for DSWAT. About every two years, we have enough vacancies to justify a SWAT selection school, usually with four to six positions to fill.

MCPD posts a vacancy announcement departmentwide. To apply, officers must be a Police Officer II (three years of experience) or Police Officer I (two years) with prior specialized military training (SEALs, etc.). Applicants must pass a PT test and a firearms qualification. Consultants from ARA/Human Factors, experts in creating job-related physical retention/accession standards for SWAT Teams, developed the PT test by interacting with the Central SWAT Team and watching what they did on a daily basis, including raids and training. ARA also helped develop standards for NASA, Metro-Dade SRT, and other specialized units.

ARA notes the following in developing the physical standards for police SWAT teams: "The essence of this procedure is to identify cut-points for the performance of certain criterion tasks below which unsafe and inefficient job performance will result in danger to life or property. Since the nature of SWAT operations is based upon a contingency model, it is generally accepted that optimal levels of fitness increase the probability of success. By expecting high levels of fitness in the applicant and incumbent population, we diminish the potential for mission failure."

ARA also makes this comment: "Consequences in failure to perform in SWAT callouts, felony arrest warrants, and narcotic search warrants are grave. Coupled with the potential for extreme liability and personal injury, standards for this position should be necessarily high. SWAT teams by definition represent an elite group of highly trained individuals. The courts have also ruled that 'there is an expectation from the community and the courts that SWAT teams represent highly trained individuals both tactically and physically.'"

Over several weeks, consultants from ARA spend a number of days observing, interviewing, and interacting with our Central SWAT Team. After conducting their research, they developed the following PT test that we administer in this order, with minimums cited for each event.

An instructor demonstrates each exercise with a focus on form and emphasizes that the students perform the movement correctly.

Candidates have advance knowledge of the components of the test, but there are no retakes, as there are no alibis in SWAT operations. The test consists of elements in Table 7.

Table 7. Montgomery County SWAT PT Qualification Standards

Activity	Standard	What the Activity Tests
Push-ups	60 (continuous)	Muscular endurance upper body
Sit-ups	45 in 1 minute	Endurance
Pull-ups	4 reps with 35-lb. weight attached (simulates weight of gear)	Power
Rope climb	35-lb. weight attached (simulates weight of gear)	Ability to traverse obstacles
Stair run	45 seconds to run up a 4-story building in full gear with 45-lb. dumbbell (simulates half the weight of 90-lb., 2-person battering ram)	Simulates rapid entry into building under exigent circumstances
3-mile run	Under 26 minutes	Cardiovascular fitness; stamina

Note: These are *minimum* physical requirements; selected candidates routinely far exceed them.

In addition to passing the PT test, applicants must also pass a tactical firearms qualification. The firearms qualification is 90%, and the course of fire is more difficult than the standard department qualification. Applicants must pass with their handgun and shotgun. They will be trained in the use of the carbine during the SWAT selection school.

Once selected to the SWAT Team, all full-time members (Central) must pass the PT test and firearms test quarterly and DSWAT officers twice a year. Failure to pass the test, absent a medically documented injury, results in removal from the team.

Typically, forty-five to fifty officers from Montgomery County apply and take the pretests. On average, about half pass the tests and attend the SWAT selection

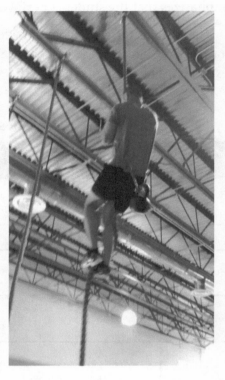

Officer Bill Mcquiggan taking a SWAT PT test involving a rope climb with a thirty-five-pound weight attached
(Courtesy of MCPD)

school. The school is also open to outside agencies, whose applicants must also pass the pretests. We have had officers from numerous local police SWAT teams, the military, and intelligence agencies attend. A usual class might have twenty-four MCPD officers and a couple from outside agencies. The three-week school is very demanding. It tests a host of factors:

- Strong emphasis on physical abilities
- Will and desire to push on when completely exhausted
- Self-initiative
- Strength of mind
- Positive attitude

- Exceptional firearms skills
- Clear understanding of tactical movements
- Ability to assess a situation quickly and make good decisions
- Ability to follow directions
- Complete assignments with attention to detail
- Leadership
- Team concept
- Ability to perform all these tasks safely with sleep deprivation

We often lose four to six people per class. Some just quit while others drop out due to injury.

A strong emphasis is placed on the need to win all the time. I use the following analogy to emphasize that point. If an NFL team goes 14-2 during the regular season, it had a great season and will make the playoffs. Our SWAT Team's season is 200 raids and barricades each year. We must go undefeated every season, every year, because the price of losing is too great.

Instructors evaluate applicants during all training phases.

Enormous emphasis is placed on physical abilities. I often tell those in the school that it doesn't impress me to be fast or to be strong; what impresses me is to be fast *and* strong. Even more important is being a team player. Occasionally, we have candidates who are the fastest or strongest and have all the required skill sets but are not team players. There is no letter "I" in the words "SWAT Team." Talented individuals have been passed over because they failed to understand this concept.

After the course, evaluators review and discuss applicant performance and make selections. Typically, out of the twenty-four students who passed the initial pretest and attended the school, evaluators select four to six.

Those selected will start a lengthy training protocol, attending numerous tactical schools. MCPD will host some schools they attend, while outside agencies host others. They also start doing tactical operations, raids, and barricades. They continue training throughout their careers and gain operational experience with time.

The members of the DSWAT Team are the future members of the full-time team, so members of Central go to great lengths to develop high-quality training venues and act as mentors.

Interesting note: On June 7, 2017, at age fifty-seven, Kamensky became the oldest active SWAT officer to pass the PT test—with twenty-one years of SWAT service. I had the honor of presenting him with the Immortal Award, a plaque recognizing his outstanding achievement.

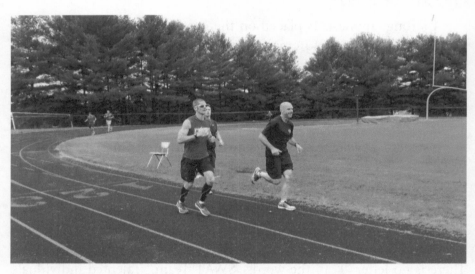

Officer Rob Kamensky, age fifty-seven (inside lane), completing a timed three-mile run for the SWAT PT test

(Courtesy of MCPD)

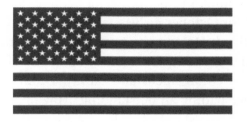

14. Retirement and Another Obstacle

Resilience

On my last day of work, September 30, 2014, I met with the SWAT Team at the SOD in the conference room to have my final words. I thanked the team for its support and all that each person had done for me during my illness. I told them I was very proud of them and wished each the best of luck.

Dillman had arranged to drive me home. I turned in my SWAT vehicle. When I got into his SUV, my son, Lawrence, was waiting in the back seat. Dillman had picked him up from school so my son could share my last day on the job. As we started to drive away from the SOD, we were escorted by about two dozen of our police motorcycle units. They all had their emergency lights on. Rather than go directly to my house, we detoured and passed in front of MCPD headquarters. Numerous officers were out front waving, standing at attention, and saluting. When we finally arrived at my house, the motorcycle units were neatly lined up at attention in front of my driveway. One APC was parked out front. The SWAT Team, Command staff, and other officers were standing by out front. Dillman arranged to have the entire event videotaped. It was impressive for others to watch and overwhelming for me personally.

What a send-off.

I had asked Dillman to be master of ceremonies at my retirement party, scheduled for October 4, 2014, at the P.B. Dye Golf Clubhouse in Ijamsville, Maryland. He and the team went to extraordinary lengths in preparing and organizing the event. More than 160 people attended, most of them law enforcement and family. Dillman made the event memorable by persuading an outstanding array of speakers to present. Stephens, who had retired to Delray Beach, Florida, several years earlier, flew up to join me—a gratifying surprise. Childs attended, along with Rizak, Arlington County Police Department, who had provided me with the referral to Childs. Retired U.S. Marine Colonel Eric Lyon delayed his deployment to Afghanistan by one day to attend. Dillman acknowledged their presence during the opening remarks.

My son, Lawrence, age twelve at the time, was asked to present an award to me. He was nervous behind the microphone and said, "I don't speak very much," and presented a framed picture of himself, a police K9 dog named Dallas, and me. He was overwhelmed with emotion and broke down in tears as he handed me the picture and said: "You are my hero." It was a touching moment; the audience gave him a standing ovation.

Upon my retirement, Dillman became SWAT commander for the MCPD, a job he had earned. He did a superb job in that position for the next four years. He was then promoted out of the unit as a lieutenant. A short time later, he was transferred back to SOD as the deputy director overseeing SWAT. He remains one of my best friends.

Three months after my retirement, on January 30, 2015, life's obstacle course took yet another turn. I suffered a stroke from the chemotherapy. I had gone to the bathroom in the early morning hours and suddenly found myself on the floor with no recollection of how I got there. I tried for several minutes to stand up, but I had no strength on the left side of my body and could not push myself up. I called out to Jayne. She noticed that the left side of my face drooped and that my speech was slurred. She immediately suspected I had suffered a stroke and called fire and rescue, which transported me to Shady Grove Medical Center for examination.

Examination confirmed that I had suffered a stroke. I was having great difficulty speaking, and my head throbbed. Jayne called Dillman and advised him of the circumstances. The SWAT Team had just done a raid, and the members were, as is their custom, having breakfast at Panera at the Fallsgrove Village Center directly across the street from the hospital.

The entire team came to see me, but I was a mess, trying unsuccessfully to talk and even drooling. Despite the circumstances, it was uplifting to see the guys. I spent two days at the hospital under observation. The doctors and staff were dedicated and thoroughly professional, but I had had it with hospitals so I called one of the SWAT guys after Jayne left and asked him to return and help sneak me out. But Jayne found out about my plans and called Dillman, who issued specific orders that nobody pick me up. Dillman, good friend that he is, was just looking after my welfare.

Finally, after half a dozen scans and tests, I was released. The stroke had hit me hard. My speech remained slurred for several months, and the left side of my face still drooped. Now, five years later, my face no longer droops. I have recovered strength on my left side, and by all appearances, no one would know I had suffered a stroke. I also had a headache that lasted several months.

As a result of the stroke, I was put on the blood thinner Xarelto, and the daily dosage of my Revlimid chemotherapy was reduced from 15 milligrams to 10 milligrams.

When Jayne picked me up from the hospital, I had a craving. As I said earlier, I have always been disciplined in my diet, so I had never had a Krispy Kreme donut. I thought: "To hell with discipline today." I got two glazed and one chocolate. Damn, they were good!

Several weeks after my stroke, Dillman stopped by to check on me. He brought me Laura Hillenbrand's *Unbroken* about Louis Zamperini, a world-class middle-distance runner who qualified for the 1936 Olympics but later, as a pilot in World War II, crashed in the ocean. After he and his companions survived a month and a half adrift in the ocean, the Japanese interned him as a prisoner of war. He endured more than two years of torture and extreme humiliation. With knowledge of the book's content, Dillman inscribed this note in it:

> "Jeff, I thought it was only appropriate that I give a true warrior a book to read about another warrior. You are the strongest individual I have ever known both physically and mentally. This book reminds me of you. You are my real-life Louie. This stroke is nothing more than another one of the many obstacles that have been put in your path that you have defeated. Keep your chin up, continue to fight and persevere like you always do. I love you my brother. God bless, Brian"

His gift and gracious words renewed my strength at a time when I was struggling to recapture my mental toughness as a result of the stroke. For me, this single act demonstrates the bond that teammates establish in SWAT environments and the value and significance of that relationship.

Cancer changed my life plans. In a perfect world, I wanted to stay in SWAT another four years, until age sixty. After retirement, I was going to work for the State Department's Antiterrorism Assistance Program. I would choose contract work at my leisure. However, frequent doctor visits, treatment, and the effects of chemotherapy no longer made that possible. Any travel I did I had to schedule during a "good week" in the chemo cycle. Overseas travel would be problematic.

Knowing my limitations, teammate Tatakis provided me the opportunity to serve as a consultant with him to the armed security element of the Lockheed Martin corporate headquarters in Bethesda, Maryland. We provided active-shooter training quarterly to the group. Ultimately, the fight to survive became too great, and after two years, reluctantly, I gave up the Lockheed Martin contract.

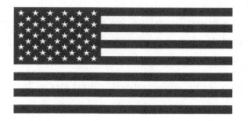

15. Remembering Our Brother

Sorrow

On August 3, 2019, I received tragic news about Ken Stephens, a talented officer who left MCPD with twenty years of service. He left to honor the wishes of his wife, Kat, to live in Delray Beach, Florida. Stephens was a martial arts instructor and began teaching classes in Florida. In 2012, he founded Tactical Combat International, a novel company that helped law enforcement agencies nationally strengthen their real-world training. Stephens also developed a women's self-defense program and achieved black-belt status in Brazilian Jiu-

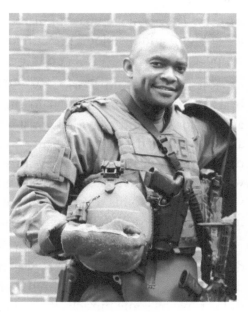

Kendrick Stephens
March 7, 1972-August 9, 2019
(Courtesy of Rob Cassels, MCPD)

Jitsu and other martial arts forms.

Kat had been diagnosed with breast cancer about a year earlier. Since Stephens and I were good buddies, he reached out to me because of my cancer experience. I had conversations with both him and his wife to provide encouragement and support and to share my own lessons.

I was shocked to learn events took a sad turn. Jason Boyer, a former police officer and martial arts instructor, was teaching a class at the Crater Criminal Justice Academy in Virginia. He invited his longtime friend Stephens to assist with teaching the class. Stephens had a seizure as he was giving a PowerPoint presentation and fell headfirst to the ground. Boyer said the strike was extremely loud. Stephens was unconscious for some time. He regained consciousness but was disoriented. He was transported to a local hospital and then to Virginia Commonwealth University Medical Center because of how serious his injuries were. Examination determined he had a fractured skull, severe bleeding of the brain, and a broken vertebra, so the medical staff rushed him into surgery. They removed part of his skull to reduce swelling, but he lost a lot of blood and his blood pressure dropped sharply. He was put on life support and was in critical condition.

Kat flew up from Florida. MCPD Officer Rob Cassels, Stephens's best friend, immediately went to the hospital. He booked a room for a week for Kat and provided constant updates. Dillman secured a van and coordinated a trip of former SWAT teammates to visit Stephens on August 7, 2019. We all knew this was likely to be the last time we would see him alive. Stephens was in a coma, and three of us at a time were allowed into his room. It was painful seeing a former teammate so incapacitated. We all talked to him with the belief that he could hear us.

Afterward, we gathered in a conference room with family, and the doctors gave a prognosis. There was no improvement over the last five days, and he was critically injured. Survival was unlikely, and even if he did survive by some miracle, it would take the constant use of machines to maintain his life. Family and doctors agreed that his quality of life was so depleted that the most prudent course of action was to let a spiritual man go to heaven.

While riding back in the van from the hospital, a collection of senior SWAT officers who had worked with Stephens reminisced about SWAT operations, including an unusual incident that became known as the hurricane breach. In September 2003, Hurricane Isabel raced up the East Coast toward the Washington, DC, region. It proved to be the most destructive, costly storm ever to strike DC. During this same time, a series of bizarre killings, which had an Alfred Hitchcock feeling, occurred in Montgomery County.

On September 17, Tristan Offiah was murdered inside his vehicle at about 2 a.m. in the 2030 block of Georgian Woods Place in Wheaton, Maryland. Investigation revealed the following: Evan Smyth told his friend James Allen Brandt he intended to rob an acquaintance named Offiah of his drugs. At Smyth's direction, Brandt drove to the location where Offiah was waiting for them. Once there, Smyth pointed out Offiah, who was sitting in his vehicle, and instructed Brandt to pull into the parking space next to Offiah's car. Smyth got his shotgun from the back seat, exited the vehicle, opened the passenger door of the other vehicle, and shot Offiah. Smyth and Brandt stole some crack cocaine in the shooting. Police found a twelve-gauge shotgun shell and a cell phone at the scene.

The next morning at 9 a.m., a citizen reported a strong odor coming from the trunk of a vehicle parked in the 2400 block of Dressler Lane. MCPD responded. Inside the vehicle they found the partially decomposed body of a man later identified as Phillip Walker. A medical examiner determined he had died of multiple stab wounds after last being seen alive on September 9.

Hurricane Isabel struck the DC region later that afternoon. Winds were strong, with a heavy downpour. After the storm started, the MCPD 911 Emergency Center received a call from a female at 12501 Arbor View Terrace in Silver Spring. She whispered, "Help me," and then the call disconnected. Uniform patrol officers responded, and when they arrived, they found both the screen door and front door ajar. The patrol units entered and found a deceased female in the basement family room. She was naked, and her head appeared to be in an unnatural position. She would later be identified as Shauntise Gill. She had last been seen alive by her mother the day before; it would later be determined she died of strangulation. A twelve-gauge shotgun was observed on a table near Gill's body. The patrol units were not sure if the suspect or suspects were still in the house. The police withdrew and formed a perimeter around the house.

They initiated an ERT callout to which SWAT responded. Mcquiggan recalls it was pouring rain when he got the page, and when he opened the trunk of his SWAT vehicle to gear up, the water just poured in.

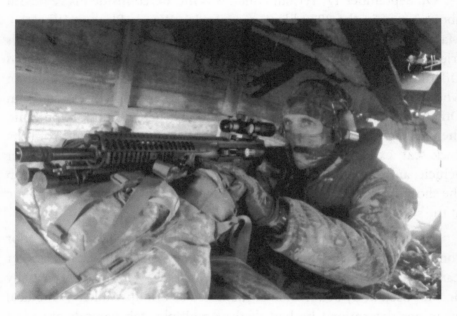

Sniper in position—fortunately, not in a ditch—during the hurricane
(Courtesy of MCPD)

Everything in the trunk immediately got soaked.

Kamensky arrived on scene and deployed as part of a two-man sniper team to cover the front of the house (Alpha side). The rain was so heavy that the arriving SWAT units decided to take shelter in an adjacent house's garage to the left (Bravo side) of the target address. SWAT attempted to contact the occupants of the house to open the garage, but no one responded.

Mcquiggan broke out a garage window, climbed through, and opened the garage door. The SWAT Team entered the garage and remained there while negotiators made phone calls to contact the target residence's occupants. There was no response, so it was quickly decided to enter and search the residence.

The sniper team covered the entry team as they approached the house. SWAT did a limited entry into the structure through the open front door. A K9 dog was deployed off lead (no leash) to search the house. The dog returned with no indication of suspects inside. The team then conducted a search with the assistance of a pole camera. One element proceeded left, and SWAT located the deceased female lying on the floor in the basement family room. A second element went to the right with Bandholz leading. He recalls proceeding through a doorway into a semi-finished recreation or basement area. The floor was initially carpeted and then turned to unfinished concrete, and he felt the floor was very slick. He cleared the room and observed what appeared to be flesh, blood, and brain matter. It was wet and plastered to the ceiling, indicating that the crime was relatively recent. On the other side of the basement, he also observed what appeared to be skull fragments and hair attached to the floor.

Finally, he saw what looked like bloody drag marks across the floor, as if someone had dragged a body out. He then realized he was slipping on the floor from brain matter on the bottom of his boots. He later put his boots into a hazmat bag and threw them out. The human tissue recovered by evidence technicians would lead to identification of a second victim, Kay Carey. We learned later that she had been killed with a shotgun. Investigation revealed that her body had been thrown into a trash dumpster in Silver Spring and then deposited in a landfill in Fredericksburg, Virginia. SWAT cleared the entire house with no other subjects located inside. SWAT then turned the crime scene over to investigators, but four SWAT officers remained behind for security in case a suspect or suspects returned. The sniper team had deployed into a ditch. They said there was twelve inches of rain in the ditch when they secured from the position. It was by far the heaviest rain and wind in which they had ever deployed.

Investigators soon learned through cell phone records and other data that all four homicide victims knew each other. Investigators quickly identified two individuals as suspects: Evan Smyth, a white male (forty), who resided at the Arbor View address that SWAT had just searched. The second subject was James Allen Brandt, a white male (twenty-seven). Investigators believed that both suspects were currently in apartment #14 at 3501 Pear Tree Court in Silver Spring. It appeared from investigator surveillance that at least three males believed to be armed were at the residence. Investigators obtained a no-knock search warrant and arrest warrants for two individuals. Hurricane Isabel's peak winds were now striking the DC region. The heavy downpour and very strong winds were causing significant property damage and power outages.

The tactical supervisor sent Craig Dickerson and me on a recon of the target address that we would use to help develop an operational plan. Dickerson was security and would lead the team to the door. My job was to assess whether we needed an explosive entry. The apartment was at ground level and had a Class-2 metal door, with a deadbolt and chain lock mechanism and a metal frame. This was standard for most older apartments at the time. It appeared to be a two-bedroom apartment with a master bath, living room, dining room, kitchen, and a hallway bath. I suggested an explosive breach on the front door because it was ideally suited for a water impulse charge, and that would provide a quick, efficient entry. I also suggested deploying flash-bangs through the bedroom windows three seconds before we initiated the explosive charge. The flash-bang 1.5-second delay would disorient any individuals inside the bedrooms as the team entered and cleared the apartment. We hoped this device would prevent the suspects from accessing weapons. We would coordinate the timing of the flash-bang deployment and subsequent explosive breach using an operational countdown. The tactical supervisor agreed to the plan. At 9:50 p.m., we executed the no-knock warrant during the height of Hurricane Isabel. The team parked the raid vans around the corner from the apartment, which let the team approach in a stealth manner. Command was concerned about the hurricane conditions during the approach because the high winds were constantly causing tree branches, loose objects, and debris to fly through the air. Ironically, as terrible as the conditions were, as we drove into the target neighborhood, the downpour stopped, the wind subsided, and a brief moment of peace ensued. It as if the eye of the hurricane passed over us at that moment, and we reached the apartment door without incident.

Dickerson, tasked with providing security to the door, placed tape over the peephole, attempted to open the door quietly, and gave a thumbs-down indicating the door was locked. We needed a breach to effect entry. Dickerson covered the door with his weapon while the assistant breacher, Winterhalter, placed the water impulse explosive charge on the door. Simultaneously, two other officers tied off the surrounding apartment doors with rope to prevent the doors from being opened by residents inside as we detonated the charge. The entry team positioned itself in a safe location, and the assistant breacher went to the rear of the stack, checking that the team was stacked low in a safe location behind the ballistic shield. I maintained control of the firing device and got a thumbs-up from the assistant breacher. I gave one last look to make sure the charge was still attached and a quick glance at the ropes to confirm the other apartments were still tied off.

I started our operational countdown on the radio: "Nine tango 13, I have control." Nine Tango 13 was my current operator's call sign, and "I have control" alerts the team that the explosive breach is imminent. Continuing the countdown: "Ready, ready." If a team member is not ready or if someone needs to abort, they must communicate the fact at this moment. "Three, two, one." At "three," we broke the bedroom windows with a Halligan bar, a forcible-entry tool that law enforcement and firefighters use. We deployed the flash-bangs through the bedroom windows. Their 1.5-second delay caused them to go off just before or as we breached the front door. A cover man protected officers breaching the windows and the subsequent distraction device deployment. On "one," I initiated the charge.

The explosive breach was successful, so the team quickly moved through the apartment, securing its occupants. At gunpoint, Bandholz took down one murder suspect, Brandt, who was in the master bedroom. McGaha assisted. The suspect was still disoriented from flash-bang effects, so they immediately handcuffed and secured him. Kamensky secured and cuffed a second subject in the hall bath. Stephens, Dickerson, and Maddox took down, secured, and cuffed the two remaining subjects in the dining/living room area. We apprehended four individuals in the apartment and turned them over to the Major Crimes Unit. Investigators charged Brandt in the murder of Offiah, the subject killed in his car with a shotgun.

We cleared the apartment and returned to our raid vans. Shortly after the team loaded into the vans, the lull in the hurricane ended, and heavy downpour and gale-force winds returned. This became known as the "hurricane breach" among the SWAT members present because of the unusual circumstances related to the raid.

Law enforcement located and arrested the second murder suspect, Smyth, the following day in Brunswick, Frederick County, Maryland. A search warrant executed on Smyth's vehicle revealed these items in his trunk: a bag containing the identification of Phillip Walker, keys, cell phone, and latex gloves. Walker's body, found in the trunk of a car, was the one causing the strong odor. Smyth was ultimately charged with the murders of Walker, Gill, Carey, and Offiah.

While returning home after visiting Stephens in August 2019, we recalled another incident in which he participated that saved the life of a young girl.

On February 27, 2009, at 12:45 p.m., the 911 Emergency Center received a report of a female on the roof of a high-rise building at 11215 Oak Leaf Drive, Silver Spring, who was threatening suicide. The complex, called The Point, consisted of a group of high-rise apartment buildings.

Charles Nicholas Riccio, a maintenance worker, was on the roof when he observed a female kneeling at the roof's edge. He thought she was going to jump so he asked her to come down with him. She shook her head and said no. Riccio remained on the roof and retreated inside a cooling tower on which he was working. Concerned about her welfare, he called the police.

The ERT responded to try to prevent the subject from jumping off the roof. It was a twenty-story high rise with a hatch that granted rooftop access. I will not reveal the subject's identity because she was a juvenile at the time. She was a distraught Asian female (seventeen) perched precariously at the roof's edge. It was a cold, blustery day. Negotiators talked to her for hours with no resolution.

I was in command of the SWAT operation. To support negotiators if the subject tried to jump, we formed a five-man IAT staged out of sight below the hatch on the twentieth floor. Each person had a specific role. Ulisney and Stephens were designated as the hands-on operators who would, if given the opportunity, grab the subject to prevent her from jumping or falling off the edge.

I picked these two men because of their skill sets. Ulisney was a former SEAL and had wrestled in high school. Stephens was a black belt in martial arts and a certified master rappeler. I felt confident that if these guys grabbed hold of her, they could immediately control her and prevent her from going off the roof. They were each secured and attached to a rappel harness.

A third officer was to assist in feeding the rope if the team was called into action. While we had no indication that the subject was armed, a fourth officer was designated "less lethal," an option to incapacitate the subject with a non-lethal weapon, and the fifth was designated "lethal force." It is always important to prepare for the unknown, as in the event the subject suddenly produced a weapon from under her clothing. We also deployed observation teams with binoculars to two adjacent high-rise buildings in an effort to gather further intelligence.

Many hours had passed. It was still very cold outside, and the wind had started to pick up. The subject now sat facing the negotiators, who were talking to her from the open hatch. She was at the very edge of the roof with a blanket around her. It was starting to get dark. Riccio, who was still in the cooling tower, was lightly clothed and cold. Negotiators advised the juvenile that Riccio would move across the roof and exit through the roof hatch. Negotiators also advised her that we would place lights just outside the hatch to provide light to the roof. During this transition, we had an opportunity to get one of our SWAT officers on the roof. Our hands-on SWAT officers, Ulisney and Stephens, had changed into civilian clothes to appear less threatening. Riccio moved across the roof and exited without incident.

Ulisney then placed the lights on the roof just outside the hatch. There was a ladder leading up to the hatch; Stephens was standing on it out of sight below Ulisney. Ulisney then engaged the subject in conversation to win her confidence. He talked about the fact that he had daughters close to her age. We developed a plan to deliver food to her, and if the opportunity presented itself, the IAT had the authority to act. The distance from the hatch to where the subject was sitting was about thirty feet. Ulisney attempted to deliver food at 8:30 p.m., but the subject refused. As soon as Ulisney moved toward her, she stood up at the roof's edge. Ulisney immediately stopped. He engaged her in conversation; soon she sat back down. Over the next few hours on several occasions, she again stood up at the roof's edge. In each instance, Ulisney calmly talked to her and got her to sit back down.

The weather was changing; a light drizzle began, winds picked up, and temperatures dropped. Of great concern: The roof had become slick so the possibility arose that a strong wind gust could blow the subject off the edge. The slick roof would also make it difficult for SWAT officers to move quickly across the roof to rescue her.

With conditions deteriorating, I re-confirmed that if the IAT saw an opportunity, they had the authority to act. I gave specific instructions about the decision to act, leaving nothing to chance, and failure was not an option. I did not want the perception that law enforcement actions caused the subject to fall or jump to her death. The stakes were high, and IAT members understood this.

The team remained staged for a couple more hours until an opportunity presented itself. The subject remained at the roof's edge and was seated facing the team. At 10:48 p.m., Ulisney saw her lie down with her eyes open, watching him. He then saw her head drop back and her eyes close. He immediately signaled to the IAT. He swiftly crossed the slick roof, followed by Stephens and other SWAT officers. Ulisney grabbed the subject with a firm hold and pulled her far away from the roof's edge, securing her by lying down on top of her. She screamed loudly. He rolled her up in the blanket with assistance from other SWAT officers so she couldn't move. He pinned her arms tightly in the blanket, safely led her down the hatch, and turned her over to uniform patrol officers. SWAT officers had remained at the ready for more than ten hours before taking action. She was transported to a local hospital for a mental evaluation to get her the help that she needed.

When negotiations fail and we use SWAT to resolve an incident, the public often views such events as an aggressive last resort. In this instance, aggressive SWAT actions saved a life and led to a peaceful outcome. Both MCPD and the Maryland Chiefs of Police Association awarded Ulisney the Silver Medal of Valor.

Stephens had a significant role in the incidents I just described: rescuing the "jumper," the search of the house in Silver Spring (scene of two homicides), and the raid we dubbed the "hurricane breach." Stephens died on August 9, 2019, at age forty-seven after being taken off life support.

The following day, I left for Lake Tahoe to visit my brother. Todd had arranged a presentation on August 13 to local law enforcement SWAT teams about the Discovery suicide bomber and DC sniper incidents. I had an opportunity to highlight the outstanding job that Stephens did during the Discovery incident. I had visited him in Delray Beach not long after his retirement, at which point he and I re-created the final beach scene of the classic 1994 movie *The Shawshank Redemption* with Morgan Freeman and Tim Robbins. Jayne filmed it on her cell phone. Stephens was very good at editing film, to my surprise, and he released the finished product on YouTube under "Kendrick Stephens Shawshank Redemption." In August 2019, I replayed it for myself to honor a true warrior.

On August 31, his wife hosted a memorial tribute at Gaithersburg High School, followed by a celebration of life at Norbeck Country Club. Hundreds of police, family, and friends attended both events. The MCPD honor guard was present to create a heartfelt tribute for a fallen teammate.

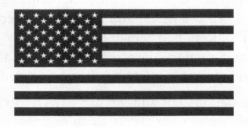

16. My Finest Hour

Perseverance

Each person faced with a life-threatening disease derives many lessons from that experience. I share some of my lessons hoping they may inspire and help others struggling with such challenges. I believe that seven factors can lead to winning a battle with a life-threatening disease.

1. Best Medical Care: I have been fortunate to have the best among my oncologist, Wallmark; Badros, who performed my stem-cell transplant; NIH assistance from Childs; and the Tufts University consultant, Comenzo—individuals recognized as among the best medical professionals in the world.

2. Patient Responsibility: While quality doctors, medical care, and treatment are critical, the patient, including myself, has numerous responsibilities to help maximize the effects of any prescribed treatment. We can all do things to help ourselves, so develop a strong mindset and a true desire to do whatever is needed to survive.

3. Positive Note and Sense of Order: I found I can start each day on a positive note and with a sense of order and build success for the rest of the day by making my bed as I did when I started to receive chemotherapy in 2012. Interestingly, Navy Admiral William H. McCraven, a SEAL for thirty-six years, reaffirmed my belief when he told the graduates during a commencement speech in 2014 at his alma mater, the University of Texas: "If you want to change the world, start by making your bed." He emphasized that this one completed task will lead to many completed tasks over the course of the day. I could not agree more.

4. *Exercise:* As noted earlier, if I can sustain exercise for thirty minutes, my head clears and the nauseous feeling from chemotherapy disappears—perhaps because endorphins associated with exercise relieve pain or stress and boost happiness, making me feel better. My mantra is that I exercise at whatever level I can on a given day.

When I went through the police academy in 1981, I set my goal on winning the Physical Training and Defensive Tactics Award because I clearly was not going to win the Academic Award. Among the various events was maximum number of push-ups and sit-ups in one set. Each Saturday at the gym, I would max out on both exercises. I was doing 1,000 sit-ups continuously and max push-ups. I was concerned that I needed more time to complete the max sit-ups because averaging forty per minute at a continuous pace would take twenty-five minutes.

The day before our final PT test, I stopped by the office of my police counselor and asked if I could start the test early because I was concerned that since this was the last class of the day, I would run out of time to complete all PT test events. I explained my dilemma, and he looked at me with a bewildered expression on his face and said, "Nyce, get out of my office!"

The next day was the PT test. The first event was max push-ups in one set. I did 232 continuous push-ups, a record that I have been told still stands. The next event was sit-ups, and it was announced it would be the maximum number of sit-ups in five minutes. Mentally, I was thrown off. I had trained for a marathon, and now the event was a sprint. I changed strategy. Instead of pacing myself at forty sit-ups per minute, I upped it to sixty a minute. It was a difficult adjustment, but I pulled it off. Upon graduation from the MCPD Academy in 1981, I was awarded the Physical Training and Defensive Tactics Award.

In sum, Table 8 indicates the range of exercise activities that I did to keep myself healthy in my fight with cancer. How much I could accomplish and how long it took me to do so varied dramatically depending on how I felt that day. The point in documenting the range is that exercise was crucial to my survival initially, recovery, and eventual remission even if it took inordinate amounts of time. The pre-illness data below is essential because had I not been as fit as I was, I most likely would not have survived the initial onslaught from multiple myeloma and amyloidosis. Last point: I have always been and continue to be an exercise fanatic; unfortunately, two rotator-cuff surgeries and being age sixty-two have led to a decline in my upper-body strength.

Table 8. Overview of Pre- and Post-Illness Exercise Regimen

Type	Walk/Run	Training Achievement
Pre-Illness—Workout Plan	Run 20 miles a week	Run 5 days, weights 5 days
Pre-Illness—Records	Best 3-mile run: 19:15 (6:25/miles) Marine Corps Marathon: <4 hrs.	Squat: 225 lbs., 51 reps in 1 set Bench press: 315 lbs., 3 reps in 1 set
Post Diagnosis—Workout Plan	Walk 15 miles a week	Walk 5 days, weights 5 days
2012—Performance after Diagnosis	Walk 15 miles a week; very slow pace, felt like I was crawling	Squat: 225 lbs., 10 reps in 1 set Bench press: 225 lbs., 10 reps in 1 set
Today—Workout Plan	Walk 25 miles per week	Walk 5 days, weights 5 days
Today—Performance	Walk slow to moderate pace at best	Squat: 225 lbs., 5 reps in 1 set Bench press: 155 lbs., 10 reps in 1 set

In my prime, I was 165 pounds at 5' 8". Today I am 155 pounds. I would like to share one workout record. I was working out in the weight room, doing squats with Ulisney, and as I mentioned, the former Navy SEAL in him always brought out the best in me. We were squatting for reps with 225 pounds. I had always been good at endurance, and my previous record was forty-five reps. I had set a goal of fifty reps. It took every ounce of strength, energy, and mindset to reach rep fifty. Upon completing my fiftieth rep, I prepared to rack the weight. Ulisney said, "What are you doing? You have one more rep." I cursed him in my mind, but he was calling me out. I completed rep fifty-one, racked the weight, and collapsed on the floor for several minutes. That moment still haunts me because often when I complete a set, I think back to that moment and force myself to do one more rep. I call it the "Ulisney factor."

5. *Nutritional Strategy:* In part, my survival depends on the foods I choose and avoid (see Chapter 11). The medical community provided some data that I lacked, but I gained most of my nutrition acumen through self-study: reading books and surfing the Internet. Years ago, I took a course from the National Strength Professionals Association that led to becoming a Certified Conditioning Specialist. That course contained a segment on exercise physiology and nutrition. In short, I educated myself to understand what I could do to reduce the effect of cancer.

6. *Support of Family and Friends:* This support has often helped me regain my strength and the resolve to confront the next challenge. When I look back on my experiences over the last eight years, I recognize and acknowledge that without this support, I would most likely never have recovered from some of these challenges.

7. *Spiritual Belief:* The last factor, and I think the most important, is that I sustained a spiritual belief. Even though, as I noted above, I am not particularly religious and rarely attend church, I do believe in a higher power and am still here because of His divine intervention. *Surviving since 2012:* Survival has meant being on chemotherapy every day of my life. As a result, I suffer from what the American Cancer Society terms "chemo brain." Doctors and researchers also call chemo brain many things, such as cancer treatment-related cognitive impairment, cancer therapy-associated change, or post-chemotherapy cognitive impairment. Most define it as a decrease in mental sharpness—that is, being unable to

remember certain things and having trouble finishing tasks or learning new skills.

The chemotherapy cycles seem to have had a cumulative effect on my body. I have lost much of the dexterity in my hands, and I often drop objects. I have mild neuropathy in my hands and feet. On occasions, I experience severe cramping in various parts of my body. I cannot multi-task, and it takes me a long time to complete any task. I am tired and sleep ten to twelve hours a day. I often have difficulty finding the right words, and on occasion, my speech is slurred. The years of medication have taken a toll, and this has been compounded by the stroke.

In the late summer of 2017, I began experiencing great fatigue and felt my cognitive abilities were declining significantly. I was numb to the world, which I attributed to the fact that I had been on chemotherapy every day of my life for almost five years. In an effort to self-correct, I went online and discovered evidence that fasting helps with chemo fog and brain repair. There is also evidence that fasting can aide in preventing cancer and may slow the spread of existing cancer. Some have speculated it may even help eliminate cancer cells. I felt I needed to do something to detox my body and improve my quality of life by reducing the chemotherapy treatment frequency. In November 2017, after talks with Wallmark, we implemented two changes.

The first change was to reduce the frequency that I was receiving chemotherapy. Typically, I would be on two chemotherapies and dexamethasone for three weeks straight and then have a fourth week off. I experimented with several combinations of reduced chemotherapy treatment under the supervision of my doctor. Ultimately, we found that a treatment of two weeks on and one week off was the best combination to reduce the frequency and keep my lab results from declining. I was close to remission but had never achieved it.

The second change was to start fasting seriously, which improves cognitive function, increases neurotrophic factors, and reduces inflammation. It also promotes autophagy—that is, it kills off old, damaged immune cells and, when the body rebounds, uses stem cells to create new healthy cells.

There is also research indicating that fasting and calorie restriction can slow and even stop the progression of cancer and tumor growth, kill cancer cells, boost the immune system, and significantly improve the effectiveness of chemotherapy and radiation treatment.

There are several suggested methods of fasting. The one I chose is termed intermittent fasting. What I have learned is that, like everyone, I get better at it the more I do it. I experimented to determine what would give me the best results. At first, I would fast three times a week for sixteen hours. I would eat all of my food in an eight-hour window. Soon I was fasting every day for sixteen hours. On one occasion, I fasted for twenty-four hours, then thirty-six, and another for forty-eight hours in an effort to figure out what worked best for me. I have reviewed about twenty research studies from credible sources such as NIH, Johns Hopkins, Mayo Clinic, Harvard, and Stanford. Ultimately, I decided to fast every day, typically for twelve to fourteen hours. I found this to be the best balance between fasting and working out because my workouts and energy levels suffered tremendously when I fasted beyond this period of time.

I followed that fasting plan for three months, and my lab results were the best they had ever been. For the first time in my life after five years of treatment, I achieved complete remission. I discussed my strategy and results with Wallmark. He concurred that there is growing evidence that fasting can assist in the treatment of cancer and suggested I continue the protocol. I have fasted every day now for twelve to fourteen hours for over two years and remain in remission.

I also shared my strategy and results with Badros. He was impressed with my lab results and said I was doing well. For some time, I visited him twice a year. Recently, he commented: "You are doing well. How about if I see you in a year?"

I visited Childs and his team at NIH in January 2019. I always like to receive their input on changes I make to my chemotherapy treatment. He said it is not uncommon to experiment with different treatment protocols for long-term chemotherapy—to see what we can reduce and still achieve effective results. He said I was rewriting the text because

I have taken them into uncharted territory, meaning that I am asking questions about protocol and treatment they have not yet had occasion to explore because so few patients with these two maladies have survived eight years. When I mentioned intermittent fasting, he was impressed with the results and said he may consider fasting himself. He suggested we only perform heart MRIs annually now because he is confident that I am in a good place.

I felt good about my visit to NIH because on a previous visit we discussed the possible need for a pacemaker. My most recent MRI showed an improvement of left ventricle function and reduced wall thickness. Images of 2D echoes showed evidence of the amyloid deposits breaking up. The amyloid breakup is very rare. NIH presented this as a case study at a conference attended by some of the world's leading cardiologists. For the moment, Childs and the NIH team feel that I do not need the pacemaker, but they continue monitoring my cardiac function.

If it were not for the outstanding medical care of my doctors, I would have been dead a long time ago. They took me from near death to remission and hope for a brighter future.

I am on a quest to cure myself. I hope that fasting will help me achieve this goal. It might sound far-fetched, but I have always believed that if I push hard in all directions, good things will happen. If I expect to survive, I will. If I expect to be cured, it can happen.

I often compare the medical advances over the last decade in treatment of my diseases to the advances I saw in SWAT over my career. When I first started in SWAT, we wore old baseball helmets painted blue. Now we have tactical ballistic helmets.

When I started, our handguns were six-shot Smith and Wesson .38-caliber revolvers, and when I left, we had Glock .45-caliber semi-automatic pistols with a 13-round magazine capacity.

Our primary weapon when I started was a short-barreled pistol grip Remington 870 shotgun, to which we attached a flashlight with a clamp. When I left, I had a Colt .223-caliber M4 equipped with an EOTech sight, a sure-fire tactical light system, and a night vision IR laser. We had come from being outfitted like Wyatt Earp in the Wild West to high-tech tactical operators.

When I started, our SWAT truck was an old FedEx-style delivery truck painted navy blue. When I left, it was a state-of-the-art multi-functional tactical support vehicle with capability ranging from weapons storage to advanced communications systems.

I use these SWAT advances as examples to make the point that there have been many medical advances as well over the last decade to treat my life-threatening diseases.

When I was diagnosed in 2012 with these maladies, both provided a prognosis of terminal. Even so, I told my doctors I would be the first to survive. Median survival rates have steadily increased over the last decade and have improved through use of novel drugs and clinical trials.

As I noted earlier, in 2012, when I was first diagnosed, a Google search showed the average life expectancy for multiple myeloma was three to four years and for undiagnosed amyloidosis eight months. I had survived two years untreated. In contrast, a Google search today indicates that the average five-year survival rate for multiple myeloma is 50%. Fewer than 10% survive ten years or more. The amyloidosis survival rate is 51% at one year, 16% at five years, and 4.7% at ten years. If I cannot cure myself, I hope a medical cure from NIH is on the horizon. Hope is a good thing that never dies for those who believe.

Given the dismal outlook we faced in 2012, I asked Jayne in 2019 what she was thinking then. Her thoughts:

Jeff and I had only been engaged one month when he received his diagnosis of late-stage multiple myeloma. Jeff had been battling numerous physical symptoms for years and had finally succumbed to seeing doctors to get answers, as his ability to pass the PT test and even do his job was plummeting. Jeff's personality characteristic of being laser focused on his mission had been both an attribute and a flaw. His huge successes in life were not due solely to talent, which he had in abundance. It had more to do with his personality and his predominant trait of throwing his whole being into whatever he wanted most. During his years as a senior member of the SWAT Team, his life and his time were solely devoted to the job. He would not miss training, he would not miss raids, he would not turn down off-duty callouts. This trait of his was, by far, what caused him to achieve what no other had. And becoming the SWAT Commander only made the trait stronger. But what made him great also made him brush aside anything else not directly pushing toward his goal. Therefore, he ignored any aches, pains, injuries, fatigue, or symptoms. When these maladies grew to such a state that they surely were going to derail his career, he reluctantly then turned his focus to them.

Unfortunately, a quick answer was not to be, as there was a laundry list of ailments he had cast aside. One by one these were diagnosed. Each time we rejoiced that we had an answer and his health would soon be restored. Yet, as each treatment brought results for that symptom, no slowdown to his physical decline appeared. He was so weak and sick that I tried in vain to get him not to take what turned out to be his final PT test. I was seriously afraid it would kill him. It almost did, but he passed on sheer determination and mindset, as his body was gravely ill. So, when the diagnosis arrived, it was bad. His numbers were so high the doctors told him they couldn't believe he was able to function at any level, never mind as a SWAT Commander.

We were told initially that he had about two years to live. My only thought at that time was to make the most of our two years. Doctors were not offering any better outcome at this stage, and things only got worse as time progressed. Jeff was given the additional abysmal diagnosis of cardiac amyloidosis, which was more life threatening than the cancer, reducing life expectancy to a year. My only thoughts were to support him, encourage him, and love him. I quickly decided that sorrow, tears, or depression would be detrimental and contrary to the way he approached problems. I never saw him flinch, cry, or complain. He matter-of-factly stated he would beat this. I had to sign on to this laser-focus on winning, no time wasted on tears.

As a follow-up to Jayne's earlier comment about being engaged one month prior to diagnosis in 2012, we were married at the Montgomery County Courthouse on February 14, 2014, under unusual circumstances. The ceremony had been scheduled for months, and Judge Eric Johnson was to perform the ceremony.

Johnson had a striking career in Montgomery County. He first served as an MCPD officer; then attorney, Office of State's Attorney; and ultimately a circuit court judge. He is a good friend; we worked out together many times in the weight room at the MCPD Academy.

As fate would have it, sixteen inches of snow fell on Montgomery County the day before the wedding. All government offices were closed the next day, including the courthouse. However, I received a phone call from Sergeant Sean Mullican, SRT deputy sheriff, who manned the courthouse, saying that the ceremony was still on and to be there.

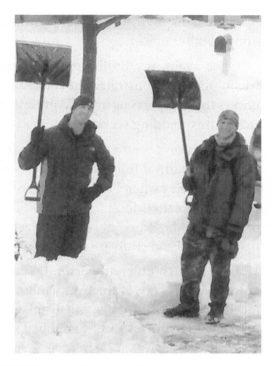

SWAT Team to the rescue—digging out my driveway
(Courtesy of Jayne Nyce)

Sean went to extraordinary lengths. He picked up Johnson in a four-wheel-drive vehicle at his house and transported him to the courthouse. He also reached out to the limited number of guests that I had invited and advised all of them that the ceremony was still on despite the weather mishap. Thanks to his effort to overcome obstacles, the event occurred.

I had not designated a specific individual as my best man. MCPD SWAT members, who are all my best friends, were present. At my request, Johnson passed my ring around to every SWAT officer present, all standing up front. He said, "Each of you is Jeff's best man." Upon receiving the ring back from Johnson, I placed the ring on Jayne's finger after we completed our vows.

Jayne's son, Brett, and my son, Lawrence, attended along with a select group of other officers.

Once again, my brothers in law enforcement and the Honorable Eric Johnson demonstrated the unbreakable bond formed among police officers that supports us in difficult times and in moments of celebration such as this wedding service.

I have always been a goal-driven individual and think it is important to pursue dreams. Mine is to be disease-free and live a normal life. I look forward to a day when I can take a deep breath and walk up a hill and not feel out of breath. I look forward to a day when I can run again. I look forward to a day when my head is clear; I am not dizzy, nauseated, and in a fog; and I can easily process data.

I am a much different person than I used to be. I was once fast and strong, had the "eye of the tiger," and was incredibly motivated to work out. I still work out daily, but it takes a greater effort physically and mentally. In many respects, I am but a shadow of the man I used to be.

Nevertheless, I still have an indefatigable will to live. I will not be deterred for there are no alibis in SWAT. I tell myself: "There is no tomorrow, only today." I remind myself: "If I didn't lose consciousness, I could have trained harder." Character isn't measured when things are great. I am at my best when challenged; the greater the odds, the greater the opportunity. Beating the odds has led to my greatest achievements and proudest moments.

Failure's not an option. Never quit, never complain, and the mission comes first. The mission is survival. Conquering cancer and amyloidosis will be my finest hour.

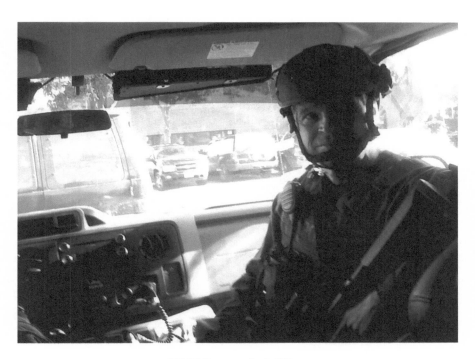

SWAT Commander Jeff Nyce
(Courtesy of MCPD)

Epilogue

In January of 2020, I had a meeting with Childs and his NIH team. They completed numerous tests and then a scheduled follow-up visit. Discussions revolved around what the future held. The results showed that I am in remission and on solid ground. Childs explained that there have been many FDA-approved treatments for the multiple myeloma and that because there are now so many options, it is likely I will remain in remission for the rest of my life. He said: "You will grow to be an old man."

There have also been medical advances in the treatment of amyloidosis. The prognosis for the future was bright in contrast to the dismal evaluation I received in 2012. These results have reinforced my hope and strong belief that I will survive and that a cure is on the horizon. I have great confidence that NIH will be the source of that cure. If not for the remarkable efforts of Childs and his NIH team, I would have perished a long time ago. I am eternally indebted and grateful.

Virginia Governor Ralph Northam, on February 21, 2020, signed legislation that creates the possibility of parole for juvenile offenders serving sentences of twenty years to life. DC sniper Lee Boyd Malvo was serving four life sentences in Virginia for the shootings. He was a juvenile when arrested. The Supreme Court dropped the pending case at the request of Malvo's attorneys. He was also sentenced to six life sentences without the possibility of parole in Maryland. The Virginia ruling does not affect the Maryland decision.

Malvo was married in early March 2020 at the Red Onion State Prison in Virginia to an unidentified bride.

On February 23, 2020, my editor, Richard Ziegfeld, tragically passed away at age seventy-one. I had great respect and admiration for him; details of his unexpected death and positive influence are described in the Acknowledgment.

In late February, my good friend Childs responded to Japan when the Diamond Princess cruise ship reported passengers with coronavirus.

He has since returned to the United States and is among those leading the charge against this virus. Despite working around the clock twenty-four hours a day, he has reached out to update me about events and check on my welfare.

A recent meeting with my oncologist, Wallmark, confirmed what I suspected. He explained that it was very important for me to follow all the recommended cautions: wearing a mask and gloves, social distancing, washing hands frequently, and remaining in the house as much as possible. The consequences could be grave if I contracted the virus. I am sixty-two years old, my immune system is weak from eight years of daily chemotherapy, and I have a severe heart condition with cardiac amyloidosis. I have always appreciated his upfront honesty. I will follow the advice of my doctor, exercise caution, and intend to survive the coronavirus outbreak.

A close friend and former neighbor, Fernando Carvajal, checked into NIH for treatment of worsening chronic lymphocytic leukemia. Upon admission, he tested positive for COVID-19. He drew strength from his past service in the U.S. Marine Corps and as a former member of MCPD DSWAT. He survived nearly a month on a ventilator and was released in April of 2020. Once again, NIH did what it does best—save lives. Amazing.

Acknowledgments

It is important that I acknowledge the efforts of Richard Ziegfeld. He served as my manuscript editor and worked with me on a host of other issues. His many years in the industry proved an invaluable resource for a first-time author.

He understood that I like to work under the team concept and that we were a team working toward a common goal. He recognized the traits that I think are critical in making our team a success: honor, integrity, commitment, dedication, and trust.

I appreciated his willingness to compromise. He was the writing subject-matter expert and had many great suggestions; I acted on the vast majority. On rare occasions, I had a different perspective and felt strongly that something needed to remain the same. We would discuss further, and if I was still passionate about an issue, he honored my perspective and did it my way. I respected him for that.

Without Richard's input, the book would not be nearly as detailed, comprehensive, or interesting as I hope the reader finds it. His input significantly enhanced the quality of my story. We both wanted to create a win-win environment that resulted in a positive experience for each. It was my hope that would occur.

Sadly, Richard died on February 23, 2020, from pneumonia. Initially, our relationship was professional and businesslike. With time, we became good friends, enjoying dinner out with our wives and others. I had great respect and admiration for him. As I mentioned previously, he displayed many characteristics and values I saw in my SWAT teammates. He was a man of honor, integrity, and trust. He was highly skillful in his craft, disciplined, and motivated; had a very strong work ethic; and understood the importance of succeeding at every task.

I learned from others—friends and family who spoke at his funeral—about the positive impact he had on so many lives. Regrettably, for all his efforts, he never saw the published book. In memory of his endeavor and as a tribute, his name is included on the cover of the book: "with Richard Ziegfeld."

Thank you, Richard Ziegfeld, for your remarkable efforts in helping me publish this book.

After Richard's shocking death, I was at a loss as to how to proceed. He had a definitive game plan and always knew what the next step would be. For several months, I pondered my next move, and then one of my best friends, George Boyce, introduced me to an acquaintance who had published several books with the help of Meredith Eaton, president of Eaton Press. I had a conversation with Matt McDarby, who had high praise for his experience with Eaton Press. I was hesitant because I am "old school" and Richard was the same, and it is my nature to be stubborn and resistant to change. My concerns quickly disappeared when I discovered Meredith was a good listener and respected how I wanted things done. She was also very good at making suggestions that would improve the quality of the book while respecting my "old school" thought process. I acted on her proposals, which I believe led to a mix of traditional and more modern concepts related to editing and publishing. I thank you, Meredith Eaton and Terri J. Huck, for your outstanding efforts in taking me over the finish line on this project.

I also want to thank Catherine Stewart, my graphic designer, who did an exceptional job on my cover design. I wanted a tactical perspective on the front cover and a medical perspective on the back, which she accomplished.

The efforts of Richard Childs, MD, Rear Admiral (RADM: Upper), in the U.S. Public Health Service Commissioned Corps, Assistant U.S. surgeon general, were extraordinary. At the height of the COVID-19 pandemic, he took the time to assist me with the back cover with his comments, provide pictures for the book, and check on my personal welfare. There are very few true difference-makers in the world, and he is certainly one of them. Our mutual friend John Rizak, a retired sergeant in the Arlington County Police Department, went to great lengths to assist me in these tasks.

My greatest thanks go to my former special operations directors and SWAT teammates, who all went to incredible lengths to help in the quest to publish this book. Chiefs of Police Darryl McSwain and Luther

Reynolds each contributed to the "praise section" of the book and had tremendous impacts on my career. Lieutenant Brian Dillman wrote the foreword and was my counterpart as the other SWAT sergeant for many years. He provided much insight with his recollections of many of the incidents described in the chapters. He coordinated and filmed the ride home on my last day on the job and served as the master of ceremonies at my retirement party.

Former Navy SEAL Rob Ulisney always motivated me in SWAT and continued to do so in my efforts to write this book. Darren Crandell stopped by my house on numerous occasions, assisting me on all fronts with anything I needed.

Rob Kamensky (the Immortal), Steve Browne, Brady Clouser, Eric Mercurio, John McGaha, Ed Clarke, Jordan Young, and Brian Dillman— all Gold Medal of Valor recipients for the suicide bomber incident at the Discovery Communications building—provided their thoughts and recollections of that event.

Bill Mcquiggan, Spiro Tatakis (the Spartan), and Paul Bandholz (wet willy) were interviewed and provided information on multiple tactical operations we did. Bill also provided numerous pictures for the book and was my designated National Geographic photographer on the last raid I ever did. Tatakis gave me direction on multiple issues related to the book.

Paul Liquorie, recently hired as chief of police in Holly Springs, North Carolina, and former Montgomery County police captain and commander of the Sixth District, provided follow-up details of a raid many years ago that left many of us who participated mystified. His explanation brought a greater level of understanding to the operation thirteen years after the incident.

Patrick Hawk, senior director of corporate security at the Discovery building, went to considerable lengths to provide information about the corporate security preparedness and crisis management plan that was implemented during the suicide bomber hostage rescue incident on September 1, 2010. Patrick shared lessons learned and improvements made several years later to further ensure the safety of Discovery's employees. An outstanding job was done the day of the incident, along with upgrades thereafter.

Officer Rob Cassels, best friend of deceased Sergeant Kendrick Stephens, helped coordinate our final trip to see Ken in the hospital before he passed away. Rob also provided a classic picture of Ken in his SWAT gear and provided details of the tragic accident that led to his death.

My brother, Todd Offenbacher, and my wife, Jayne, assisted with numerous aspects of this book, including reviewing chapters for clarity and providing input on various experiences and thoughts on marketing the book.

I wrote this book for one reason: to honor the Montgomery County Police Department and our SWAT team and to share my tactical and medical journey with my team, family, and friends. In these troubled times, I wanted to reaffirm that there are an infinite number of good cops out there, and I had the privilege of working with many of them in our department.

Jeff Nyce
July 2020

Appendix 1: Cast of Characters

Incident	Suspects
Snipers	John Allen Muhammad Lee Boyd Malvo
Discovery Suicide Bomber	James Jae Lee
Serial Bank Robbers	Miquel Morrow And 8 others
Hells Angels Motorcycle Club	Lewis J. Hall
Officer Down	Nicholas Omar Banks
Hurricane Breach Murder Suspects	Evan Smyth James Allen Brandt

Name	Last Rank	Organization; Relation	Incident
Drew Tracy	Assistant Chief	MCPD SOD	• DC Snipers
Darryl McSwain	Assistant Chief	MCPD SOD	• Discovery
Luther Reynolds	Assistant Chief	MCPD SOD	• Authorized creation of Code RED Teams
Brian Dillman	Lt.	MCPD	• Discovery • Hurricane Breach
Rob Kamensky	Sgt.	MCPD	• Discovery • Hurricane Breach
Rob Ulisney	Sgt.	MCPD	• Discovery • Jumper
Brady Clouser	Sgt.	MCPD	• Discovery
Dave Reed	Sgt.	MCPD	• Discovery
Paul Bandholz	Sgt.	MCPD	• DC Snipers • Hurricane Breach • Serial Bank Robbers
Kendrick Stephens	Sgt.	MCPD	• Discovery • Hurricane Breach • Jumper
Kevin Reese	Sgt.	MCPD	• Officer Down
Jayne Nyce	Corporal	MCPD, family	• Stem-Cell Transplant
Dave Thomas	PO3	MCPD SOD	• DC Snipers • Serial Bank Robbers

Name	Last Rank	Organization; Relation	Incident
John McGaha	PO3	MCPD	• Sniper • Discovery • Hells Angels
Steve Browne	PO3	MCPD	• Discovery • Hells Angels • Serial Bank Robbers
Bill Mcquiggan	PO3	MCPD	• State Dept. • Hurricane Breach
Spiro Tatakis	PO3	MCPD	• Discovery • State Dept.
Darren Crandell	Sgt.	MCPD	• Officer Down • Discovery
Eric Mercurio	PO3	MCPD	• Discovery
Edward Clarke	PO3	MCPD	• Discovery
Jordan Young	PO3	MCPD	• Discovery • Fooling Observers
Dan Maddox	PO3	MCPD	• DC Snipers • Hurricane Breach
Craig Dickerson	PO3	MCPD	• Hurricane Breach
Edward Paden	PO3	MCPD	• Discovery
John Wilkes	PO3	MCPD	• Discovery
Bill Seidel	PO3	MCPD	• Officer Down

Name	Last Rank	Organization; Relation	Incident
Reinold Winterhalter	PO3	MCPD	• Hells Angels • Remembering Our Brother
Sean Mullican	Lt.	MC Sheriff's Office	Discovery Finest Hour
Keith Runk	Lt.	MSP	DC Snipers Discovery
Chuck Pierce	Supervisor.	FBI HRT	DC Snipers
William McCarthy		FBI HRT	DC Snipers
Paul Jaskot		FBI HRT	DC Snipers
Neil Darnell		FBI HRT	DC Snipers
John Rizak	Sgt.	Arlington County PD	Referral to friend Richard Childs MD
Kevin Frazier	Capt.	Montgomery County Bomb Squad	Discovery
Mike Redding	Capt.	Montgomery County Bomb Squad	Discovery
Patrick Hawk	Security Director	Discovery HQ	Discovery
Lawrence T. Nyce	N/A	Family, son	Last Raid
Todd Offenbacher	N/A	Family, brother	Fooling Observers

Name	Last Rank	Organization; Relation	Incident
Richard Childs	MD; Rear Adm. (RADM: Upper), Assistant U.S. Surgeon General	NIH NHLBI	Evaluation of treatment plans; cardiology review
John Wallmark	MD	Maryland Oncology	Diagnosis of cancer and amyloidosis
Ashraf Badros	MD	MMC	Stem-Cell Transplant
Eric Johnson	Judge	MC Circuit Court	Finest Hour
Alan Brosnan	Commander	New Zealand SAS	Trained MCPD Explosive Breaching Element

Appendix 2: Medical Terms

Term/Drug	Description
Amyloidosis	Most common type is named AL. Caused by the deposition of light chain proteins produced by plasma cells in different disease states
ALT	Enzyme that helps a liver absorb protein more readily, which affects metabolism. If a liver is inflamed, it releases ALT in the bloodstream, prompting high ALT readings. ALT tests help evaluate liver health and diagnose liver problems.
AST	AST is another enzyme for which test numbers should be low. When the liver is damaged, AST numbers rise.
Bone marrow biopsy	Extracts a bone marrow tissue sample using a small needle placed into the bone. Checks on whether the body is producing healthy blood cells.
Chemo brain or fog	A side effect of chemotherapy. Causes thinking and memory problems such as confusion, being disorganized, difficulty concentrating, short attention span
Congo red	An organic compound. Water-soluble, yielding a red colloidal solution; its solubility is greater in organic solvents. However, use of Congo red has long been abandoned, primarily because of its carcinogenic properties.
Misfolded proteins	Normally, protein structures hold into a precise 3D shape. When they misfold, the aberrant structures become nonfunctional and lead to disorders such as Parkinson's, Alzheimer's, Huntington's, and Creutzfeldt-Jakob diseases.
MRI	Uses powerful magnets, radio waves, and a computer to make detailed pictures of body organs and tissues. Monitors how well patients have responded to treatment.

Term/Drug	Description
Multiple myeloma	Cancer of plasma cells that are a type of white blood cell responsible for providing antibodies. In multiple myeloma, collections of abnormal plasma cells accumulate in the bone marrow and interfere with production of normal blood cells. Bone fractures are common with multiple myeloma because it weakens and thins bones.
Neuropathy	Result of nerve damage outside the brain. Prompts tingling, prickling, or numbness in extremities. Caused by chemotherapy, diabetes, inflammation, etc.
Stem-cell transplant	Replaces damaged stem cells with healthy cells. Before the fact, chemotherapy kills malfunctioning bone marrow. Healthy cells may come from patient (autologous) or outside sources (e.g., umbilical cord or adult stem cells). Significant controversy attends use of umbilical-cord cells, which are usually harvested via abortion.

Appendix 3:

Drugs Taken to Survive Cancer

Term/Drug	Status	Description
Cytoxan	Generic	Anti-cancer chemotherapy.
Dexamethasone	Generic	An anti-inflammatory medication used as a treatment for a variety of cancers, such as leukemia, lymphoma, and multiple myeloma. Treats nausea and vomiting associated with some chemotherapy drugs.
Doxycycline	Generic	Antibiotic used to minimize amyloid deposits
Melphalan	Generic	Treats multiple myeloma and other forms of cancer by reducing the uncontrolled cell division that characterizes cancer. Chemotherapy.
Neupogen	Generic	Manufactured protein to stimulate growth of white blood cells when cancer or chemotherapy administered for bone marrow transplant preparation disrupts the creation of white blood cells.
Ninlaro	Brand name	Chemotherapy specific to multiple myeloma; slows or stops the growth of cancer cells.
Revlimed	Brand name	Form of chemotherapy used to treat multiple myeloma.
Velcade	Brand name	Used to treat multiple myeloma; interferes with cancer-cell growth. Chemotherapy.
Xarelto	Brand name	Treats deep vein thrombosis (type of blood clot); thins the blood.

Credits and permissions

- Page 108: Joel Haley, Associate Director, EMRTC, New Mexico T/E Illustration, Confirmed Person-Borne Improvised Explosive Device, New Mexico Tech, Energetic Materials and Testing Center, 2008

Photo credits by individual or organization name

- Pages 34, 35, 36: Law enforcement sources
- Pages 47, 50, 53, 54, 61, 62, 70, 72, 74, 106, 113, 135, 156, 160, 162, 170, 189: Montgomery County Police Department (MCPD) sources
- Page 78: Steve Matthews, MCPD
- Pages 124, 125: Bill Mcquiggan, MCPD
- Page 133 and back cover: Richard Childs, MD, Rear Admiral (RADM: Upper), United States Public Health Commissioned Corps, Assistant Surgeon General
- Page 133 and back cover: National Institutes of Health
- Pages 142, 154, 187, 227, "About the Author": Jayne Nyce, MCPD
- Pages 150, 151: Court Leve
- Page 167: Rob Cassels, MCPD

Bibliography

"Anatomy of a Takedown: The Washington Sniper." London: Wall to Wall Television, 2009.

"The Blood and Marrow Transplant Program and You: A Guide for Recipients of Autologous Transplants and Their Families." Baltimore: University of Maryland Medical System and University of Maryland Marlene and Stewart Greenebaum Cancer Center, n.d.

"Development of Job-Related Physical Performance Standards for the Montgomery County Police Special Weapons and Tactics Team (SWAT)." Albuquerque, NM: ARA/Human Factors, 1992.

"Directive Function Code 131: Use of Force" in Montgomery County Police Field Operations Manual. Rockville, MD: Montgomery County Police Department, 1998.

"Directive Function Code 950: Emergency Response to Hostage Barricade Situations and All Life- Threatening Situations" in Montgomery County Police Field Operations Manual. Rockville, MD: Montgomery County Police Department, 2003.

"Initial Law Enforcement Response to Suicide Bombing Attacks (IERSBA) Training Support Package." Socorro, NM: New Mexico Tech Energetic Materials Research and Testing Center, 2009.

Servan-Schrieber, David (MD, PhD). Anticancer: A New Way of Life. New York: Viking, 2007.

"Tactical Section Standard Operating Procedures." Rockville, MD: Montgomery County Police Department, 2008.

End Notes

Chapter 1: Snipers

1   MCPD SWAT PT Standards: ARA/Human Factors. Development of Job-Related Physical Performance Standards for the Montgomery County Police Special Weapons and Tactics Team (SWAT), 1992. p. 20.

2   Shooting of Buchanan: MCPD Police report, p. 20.

3   Shooting of Walekar: MCPD Police report, p. 21.

4   Protecting motorcade: conversation Drew Tracy, p. 21.

5   Shooting of Ramos: MCPD police report, p. 21.

6   Shooting of Rivera: MCPD police report, p. 21.

7   Shooting of Charlot: MCPD police Radio, p. 22.

8   Shooting Michaels Store: MCPD police report, p. 22.

9   Shooting of Martin: MCPD police report, p. 22.

10   Identify weapon as: .223: ATF p. 22.

11   Shooting of Seawell: Anatomy of a Takedown the Washington Sniper Documentary I did for Discovery Channel (wall to wall – A Shedmedia Company), p. 23.

12   Shooting of Brown: Anatomy of a Takedown the Washington Sniper Documentary I did for Discovery Channel (wall to wall – A Shedmedia Company), p. 26.

13   Shooting of Myers: Anatomy of a Takedown the Washington Sniper Documentary I did for Discovery Channel (wall to wall – A Shedmedia Company), p. 26.

14   Shooting of Bridges: Anatomy of Takedown the Washington Sniper Documentary I did for Discovery Channel (wall to wall – A Shedmedia Company, p. 27.

15   Shooting of Franklin: Anatomy of a Takedown the Washington Sniper Documentary I did for Discovery Channel (wall to wall – A Shedmedia Company), p. 27.

16 Shooting of Hopper: Anatomy of a Takedown the Washington Sniper Documentary I did for Discovery Channel (wall to wall – A Shedmedia Company), p. 27.

17 Shooting of Johnson: Anatomy of a Takedown the Washington Sniper Documentary I did for Discovery Channel (wall to wall – A Shedmedia Company), p. 27.

18 ID of Malvo, Mohammad suspect vehicle: MCPD police reports (task force), p. 28.

19 Donahoe's actions: MCPD police reports (task force), p. 28.

20 Bandhotz actions: interview, p. 30.

21 IRA: Tracy advised, p. 35.

22 Finding Bushmaster Rifle: Task Force Evidence Technicians (MCPD report,) p. 36.

23 Sentencing Malvo, Mohamad: Washington Post, 10/14/19, p. 37.

24 Medical Reports: Doctor Wallmark's online patient portal, p. 38.

Chapter 2: Hells Angels

25 Suspect Hall: MCPD SWAT raid report and ATF OP's briefing and follow-up intel, Washington Post 07/31/03, Michael Amon, p. 39, 42.

26 Taser: MCPD Instructors lesson plan, p. 42.

27 Takedown of Hall: interview MCPD SWAT officer McGaha, p. 41-42.

Chapter 3: Serial Bank Robbers

28 Details of the 6 Bank Serial Bank robberies: Briefs from MCPD task force to apprehend suspects, Op's brief from U.S Marshal service, MCPD SWAT raid report, p. 44-46.

29 Comments of video taken by cameraman "Scott" of WTTG: featured on John Walsh's "America's Most Wanted", p. 45.

30 Comments FBI agent Kinnally: Washington Times, 08/04/04, p. 52.

31 Patton quote; "Don't tell people how to do things, tell them what

to do and let them surprise you with their results," was familiar quote with as kid, reaffirmed BrainyQuote, p. 52.

Chapter 4: State Department Raid

32 Details of raid: MCPD SWAT raid report, OP's brief by Federal Investigators, p 54.

33 Details of other structure: Bill Mcquiggan interview, p 55-56.

34 Details learned 13 years later: Paul Liquorie, Interview p. 56-57.

Chapter 5: Officer Down

35 Details of incident to include identity of suspect Banks: MCPD incident report, MCPD SWAT ERT Callout report, p. 58-64.

Chapter 6: Discovery Suicide Bomber

36 Details of incident: ERT SWAT Callout Report, MCPD Major Crimes report, Montgomery County Bomb Tech/ Fire Marshals report, chronological account of minutes from Command bus log. Audio recording of incident from MCPD, Initial Law Enforcement Response to Suicide Bombing Attacks Training Support Package, 2009. Copyright NMT/EMRTC 2008. p. 65-116.

37 Certified Bomb Techs: Montgomery County Fire Rescue Bomb and Arson Unit, p. 66.

38 Madrid train bombings: Wikipedia p. 67.

39 London subway bombings: Wikipedia p.67.

40 Mumbai terrorist attacks: Wikipedia p. 67.

41 N.Y. City car bomb: Wikipedia p. 68.

42 Beslan school takeover: Wikipedia p. 69.

43 Discovery 1.5 billion subscriber's, 180 countries: Discovery. corporate.discovery.com, 06/02/10, p 69.

44 Hostages; Fisher, Wood, McNulty: MCPD police report, p. 71.

45 911 caller: MCPD recording, p. 71.

46 MCPD radio Communications: MCPD recording, p. 71-74

47 NCR building side designations: Wikipedia, p. 76.

48 James Lee activist beliefs: SaveThePlanetProtest.com/protest.htm, p. 78-79.

49 James Lee prior arrests: MCPD police report, p. 79.

50 Jackie Love security officer: personal conversation, 3 years after incident, p. 79.

51 Operation Eastern Exit: interview SEAL Rob Ulisney p. 80.

52 Clock and Distance Sniper: Wikipedia, p. 80.

53 Evacuation 1900 employees, 50 kids: conversation with Patrick Hawk, Director Security Discovery H.Q., MCPD police report, p. 82.

54 Unattended rolling briefcase: personal conversation on scene with R.J. Porath, FBI, SWAT, p. 82.

55 MCPD Directive Function Code: 131, Use of Force: MCPD Field Operations Manual, p. 83.

56 Montgomery County Fire Rescue Bomb and Arson Unit assessment of PIED, p. 84-85.

57 Hurricane glass: Glass.com, p. 86.

58 Mil dot reticle: Leupold.com, p. 87.

59 Rescue Captain Phillips: Wikipedia, p. 88.

Chapter 7: Discovery Hostage Rescue

60 Details of incident: ERT SWAT Callout Report, MCPD Major Crimes report, Montgomery County Bomb Tech Fire Recue Bomb and Arson unit report, chronological account of minutes from Command bus log. Audio recording of incident from MCPD, p. 91-101.

61 Wilkes negotiator: personal conversation I had with him after incident, p. 92-93.

62 Negotiations dialogue: MCPD Command bus log, p. 93-96.

63 Mercurio actions: Interview, p. 96-102.

64 Peltor tactical headsets: OpticsPlanet.com, p. 96.

65 Dillman Discovery assault: Interview, p. 96-100.

66 McGaha Discovery assault: Interview, p. 98.

67 Stephens Discovery assault: Interview after incident, p. 98-99.

68 Reed Discovery assault: Interview, p. 98-101.

69 Clarke Discovery assault: personal conversation after incident, p. 99.

70 Browne Discovery assault: interview, p. 99.

71 Young Discovery assault: personal conversation after incident, p. 99.

72 Clouser Discovery assault: personal conversation after incident, p. 99-100.

73 Tatakis Discovery assault: personal conversation after incident, p. 100-101.

74 Mapp gas: Wikipedia, p.100.

Chapter 8: Discovery Aftermath

75 Frazier coordination bomb squad activities: Numerous personal conversations and presentations given through the U.S.A. together, p. 104-105.

76 Pan Disrupter: Techlink p. 104.

77 Final assessment PBIED: FBI Explosives Laboratory Quantico, Va., p. 105-106.

78 Divine Intervention: Quote by Samuel Jackson in 1994 movie Pulp Fiction directed by Quentin Tarantino, p. 107.

79 PBIED response protocol: New Mexico Tech PBIED chart, p. 108-109.

80 Review .223 round effectiveness: FBI ballistic experts recommendation p. 110.

81 Barrel twist: Berger Bullets, p. 110.

82 Solution LWRC with Nightforce scope: interview with Kamensky,

MCPD firearms SME, p. 110.

83 Death before Dishonor: expression USMC p. 111.

84 Discovery Security response: interview Patrick Hawke, SR. Director Corporate Security, After action report; Corporate Security Preparedness and Crisis Management, September 1st, 2010. Patrick Hawk, Sr. Director of Corporate Security, David Sterner, Manager of Corporate Security, p. 112-114.

85 Congressional Badge of Bravery details: Office of Justice Programs (BJA), p. 115.

Chapter 9: Diagnosis Terminal

86 Tests in effort to determine illness to include hear biopsy: Washington Hospital Center, D.C., p. 117-118.

87 Amyloidosis details: Mayo clinic, patient care and health info, p. 118.

88 Multiple Myeloma details: Mayo clinic, patient care and health info p. 118.

89 Diagnosis of compression fracture back: Wallmark MD, after reviewing requested exam with radiologist, p. 118.

90 Treatment plan: Developed by Wallmark, p. 119.

Chapter 10: The Last Raid

91 Threat matrix for search warrants to determine if SWAT needed: MCPD Field operations Manual, p. 121.

92 Duval in movie Apocalypse Now: 1979 epic war film, produced by Francis Ford Coppala, p. 124.

93 Chemotherapy cycle details: Wallmark, MD, p. 128.

Chapter 11: Stem Cell Transplant

94 Childs background: NIH government website, p. 131-132.

95 Rizak discussing Ebola by Childs response and team building

interview, p. 133-134.

96 Comenzo SME amyloidosis Tuft University: conversation by phone, p. 133-134.

97 Autologous stem cell transplant: University of Maryland Marlene and Stewart Greenbaum Cancer Center guide for recipients of autologous transplants and their families, p. 134-135.

98 Boston Marathon bombings: Wikipedia, p. 137.

99 Corrective nutritional actions table 2 to counter medical challenges: Healthline, Anti Cancer A New way of Life, David Servan-Schreiber, MD, PhD, VERYWELL family food and Nutrition, LIVESTRONG, p. 138-139.

100 Stem cell preparation, aftermath: Badros, MD, p. 142-144.

101 Colonel Kilgore dress up: Duval in movie Apocalypse Now: 1979 epic war film, produced By Francis Ford Coppala, p. 144-145.

102 Engraftment phase: University of Maryland Marlene and Stewart Greenbaum Cancer Center guide for recipients of autologous transplants and their families, p. 147.

103 Post transplant safety precautions: University of Maryland Marlene and Stewart Greenbaum Cancer Center guide for recipients of autologous transplants and their families, p. 148.

Chapter 12: Fooling the Trained Observers

104 "Yippee Ki Yea", quote from 1998 movie Die Hard, directed by John McTiernan, p. 152.

105 Todd Offenbacher background: interview, p. 151-152.

106 Steve Lockshin, details aircraft, boat: phone interview, p. 153-154.

107 Bone marrow biopsy: performed by Wallmark, MD, p. 155.

Chapter 13: SWAT Selection Standards

108 Development MCPD SWAT PT standards: ARA/Human factors, 1992, p. 158-159.

Chapter 14: Retirement and Another Obstacle

109 Medical confirmation of stroke: Shady Grove Adventist Hospital, Rockville, Md., p. 165.

110 Dillman presentation of book: Unbroken, Laura Hillenbrand, p. 165-166.

111 Lockheed Martin H.Q. active shooter training: Tatakis p. 166.

Chapter 15: Remembering our Brother

112 Tactical Combat International: Website Tactical Combat International, p. 167.

113 Details of Kendrick Stephens fall and death: personal conversations with Jason Boyer and Rob Cassels, I was present when prognosis was given to family and friends at hospital, p. 168.

114 Details of events leading to "hurricane breach" incident: MCPD SWAT raid report, MCPD reports, interviews with Bandholtz, Dillman, Mcquiggan, Kamensky, p. 169-174.

115 Hurricane Isabel: Wikipedia, p. 169.

116 Details of incident at high-rise complex The Point: MCPD ERT callout report, MCPD Incident Police report, interview Ulisney, p. 174-177.

117 Shawshank Redemption recreated last scene on beach: 1994 classic movie Shawshank Redemption with Morgan Freeman and Tim Robbins. Jayne filmed it on cell phone. Ken was very good at editing film, and to my surprise released the finished product on YouTube under "Kendrick Stephens Shawshank", p. 177.

Chapter 16: My Finest Hour

118 Navy Admiral William H. McCraven (SEAL), importance of making your bed: website Inc.com, p. 178-179.

119 Endorphins: Medical News Today article, 02/06/18, p. 179.

120 Chemo brain: American Cancer Society 06/09/16, Mayo clinic, p. 181-182.

121 Fasting and cancer: Medical News Today, 01/14/19, NIH 05/22/19, Verywell Health 12/08/19, Mark Mattson, John Hopkins University, 01/01/20, Mayo clinic, Stanford University, Harvard University, USC News 03/17/17, p. 182-183.

122 Amyloidosis survival rate: NIH, NCBI S. Sachchithanantham, 2015, Medscape, 05/09/19, ncbi.nlm.nih.gov/pmc/articles/PMC3946702, 02/15, p. 185.

123 Multiple myeloma survival rate: National Cancer Institute, Everyday Health multiple Myeloma, p. 185.

124 "Eye of the Tiger": phrase made popular by song artist Survivor p. 188.

Epilogue:

125 Malvo, Source CBS News, Feb 26, Melissa Quinn, p. 191.

126 Malvo, Fox News, March 10, 2020, Louis Casiano, p. 191.

127 Carvajal, Fernando, April 22, 2020, personal interview p. 192.

Index

Transplant unit, 142, 144, 145

Travolta, John, 107

U

U.S. Marshals Service, 23, 45

Ulisney, Rob, 66, 67, 80, 131, 175, 176, 177, 181, 198

University of Maryland Medical Center (UMMC), 16, 119, 133, 134, 135

University of Texas, 179

V

Virginia Commonwealth University Medical Center, 168

W

Walekar, Premakuar, 20, 21

Walker, Phillip, 169, 174

Wallmark, Dr. John, 38, 127, 134, 138, 178, 182, 183, 192

Walsh, John, 17, 45

Water-impulse charge 47, 49, 51, 60, 171

Whalen, Sgt., 59

White box truck, 21, 27

White van, 27, 29

White-blood cell count, 136, 139, 140, 146, 147

Wilkes, John, 92, 93, 94, 95, 96, 199

Winterhalter, Reinold, 41, 173, 200

Wood, Christopher Brooks, 71

Y

Young, Jordan, 99, 115, 149, 195

Z

Zamperini, Louis, 12, 165

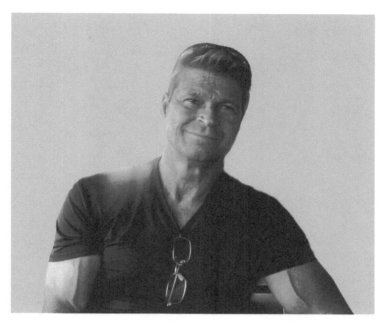

Photo Credit: Jayne Nyce

About the Author

JEFF NYCE is a former member of the Montgomery County, Maryland, Department of Police, Special Weapons and Tactics Team, known as SWAT. In his many years in SWAT, he participated in approximately 4,500 tactical operations, including the takedown of the DC snipers, the Discovery headquarters suicide bomber hostage rescue incident, and the capture of a violent group of serial bank robbers featured on America's Most Wanted.

He served as an operator, team leader, and commander. His thirty years in SWAT was the longest in the history of the team. He was struck down at the height of his career by two diseases deemed terminal at the time. Despite coding during a stem-cell transplant in 2013 and suffering a stroke in 2015, he has persevered. Eight years post-diagnosis, he is in remission and by all medical accounts has defied the odds. This is the story of how his years in SWAT prepared him for the greatest fight of his life.

Made in United States
Troutdale, OR
10/02/2024

23315519R00137